No Perfect Birth

Anthropology of Well-Being
Individual, Community, Society

Series Editor: Ben G. Blount, PhD (SocioEcological Informatics)

Mission Statement

Well-being is central and important in people's daily lives and life history. This book series brings about understanding of what the complex concepts of well-being include. The concepts of quality of life, life satisfaction, and happiness will be explored and viewed at the individual level, the community level, and the level of society. The series encourages and promotes research into the concept of well-being, how it appears to be defined culturally, and how it is utilized across levels and across different social, economic, and ethnic groups. Understandings of how well-being promotes stability and resilience will also be critical to advances in understanding, as well as how well-being can be implemented as a goal in resisting vulnerabilities and in adaptation. Series books include monographs and edited collections by a range of academics, from rising scholars to experts in relevant fields.

Advisory Board Members

Steven Jacob, Kathleen Galvin, Carlos Garcia-Quijano, Cynthia Isenhour, and Richard Pollnac

Recent Titles in the Series

No Perfect Birth: Trauma and Obstetric Care in the Rural United States, by Kristin Haltinner

Love and its Entanglements among the Enxet of Paraguay: Social and Kinship Relations within a Market Economy, by Stephen Kidd

Care Work and Medical Travel: Exploring the Emotional Dimensions of Caring on the Move, by Cecilia Vindrola-Padros

Being Ethical among Vezo People: Fisheries, Livelihoods, and Conservation in Madagascar, by Frank Muttenzer

Tourism and Maternal Health: Customs, Beliefs, and Everyday Practices, by Allison Cantor

No Perfect Birth

Trauma and Obstetric Care in the Rural United States

Kristin Haltinner

LEXINGTON BOOKS
Lanham • Boulder • New York • London

Published by Lexington Books
An imprint of The Rowman & Littlefield Publishing Group, Inc.
4501 Forbes Boulevard, Suite 200, Lanham, Maryland 20706
www.rowman.com

6 Tinworth Street, London SE11 5AL, United Kingdom

British Library Cataloguing in Publication Information Available

Library of Congress Cataloging-in-Publication Data

Names: Haltinner, Kristin, author.
Title: No perfect birth : trauma and obstetric care in the rural United States / Kristin
    Haltinner.
Description: Lanham : Lexington Books, [2021] | Series: Anthropology of well-being:
    individual, community, society | Includes bibliographical references and index.
Identifiers: LCCN 2021017945 (print) | LCCN 2021017946 (ebook) |
    ISBN 9781793643957 (cloth) | ISBN 9781793643940 (ebook)
Subjects: LCSH: Maternal health services—United States. | Childbirth—United States. |
    Obstetrics—United States. | Obstetrics—Social aspects—United States.
Classification: LCC RG960 .H27 2021 (print) | LCC RG960 (ebook) |
    DDC 362.198200973—dc23
LC record available at https://lccn.loc.gov/2021017945
LC ebook record available at https://lccn.loc.gov/2021017946

To Ethan, Garrett, and Young

Contents

Acknowledgments

To my parents, Joanna and Dennis Haltinner, I would not be here without you. I am forever indebted to the work you did to make my career is possible. From all of my being, thank you.

To Ashley Kerr. I still cannot believe that you were willing to read this entire book, multiple times, to help me get it right. Beyond that, the litany of texts and conversations. You are an amazing friend and colleague.

To Leanna Keleher and Sarah Deming. This would not have happened without you. Not only because you helped with the data collection and analysis. Truth be told, there were many times I didn't want to continue working on this project. Thinking of the two of you made it possible for me to power through. You are both among the smartest, most dedicated, most thoughtful people I've ever met. I'm so grateful you gave your time and effort to this project. I can't wait to call you both "Dr." in the future.

To Vania Brightman. The idea to study traumatic births was your brain baby. I hope that you, too, find time to continue this important scholarship and I'm so thankful you entrusted me to do so as well.

To my fellow sociologists, Ryanne Pilgeram, Debb Thorne, Leontina Hormel, and Dilshani Sarathchandra. I couldn't have done this without the best colleagues in the world. We are a fierce team, and I wouldn't want to educate, grow, learn, and struggle with any other group of people.

To Mark Warner. Thank you for having the insight and consideration to bend routines so that I could heal after Ethan's birth. To Brian Wolf and Sean Quinlan. Thank you for supporting and investing in me and my work.

To Aleksandra Hollingshead and Cynthia Moore. Thank you for supporting my sanity while I attempted to write a book during a pandemic. Our "walks," texts, and calls gave me the mental space to complete this project.

To Young Clevenger. Thank you for your support, encouragement, and for providing good distraction during the writing of this book. You are an amazing young man and I'm so grateful to get to be your bonus/stepmom.

To Garrett Clevenger. Well, I did it. Thanks to you. Writing a book during a global pandemic with kids at home isn't easy. But it was possible because of you. Thank you for your emotional support but also the time, space, and routines you helped me organize to make this possible.

To my son, Ethan Clevinner. My darling boy. You are such a gift. My life would be incomplete without you and I'm so grateful for our relationship. I look forward to a lifetime of watching you grow, learn, create, and change discourses.

To the women who shared their stories. I am forever in your debt. Thank you for your willingness to trust me with your experiences. I hope I've done you justice.

Introduction

Traumatic Childbirth in Springfield and Greenfield

When I was thirty-six weeks pregnant, I went into preterm labor. My earliest memory of my time in the hospital was lying in a bed strapped with monitors, the head nurse, Brenda,[1] talking to me. The contractions were fierce and frequent, but I was not in active labor. Brenda, an experienced nurse, called the doctor and told him to get to the hospital as quickly as possible.

The next thing I remember, I was in the elevator on a gurney being wheeled into the operating room for an emergency cesarean. I had only been in the hospital for 30 minutes. The anesthesiologist administered a numbing agent to my back. They started the surgery. A few minutes later, Dr. Fischer pulled my son from my body and took him to an incubator to be examined. Dr. Fischer continued to stitch up the hole in my abdomen. At the time, I did not know what was transpiring, but I could sense the panic in the room. Eventually, the medical staff brought him to my head for a quick photo and then whisked him away.

Later, Dr. Fischer explained what happened. When he sliced into my uterus, he saw it was black. My son was floating in a sack filled with meconium, the black, tar-like early stool of babies. This is not normal and indicates a serious problem. At subsequent visits with the doctor, I learned my placenta was riddled with blood clots, and my son was not getting adequate sustenance. As a result, he was very small for his gestational age, weighing only three and a half pounds.

After the postoperation recovery time, I was moved to a birth suite. My son, however, had to stay in the nursery. The nurses made it an isolation unit for him so that he would not experience any undue stimulation. Meanwhile, I lay in my bed down the hall. I was receiving magnesium sulfate to reduce my blood pressure, and it left me feeling weak and nauseous. I remember long hours alone in my hospital room reading parenting books and trying to select a name for my son. We finally settled on Ethan. It means strong.

On the third day, Ethan's condition had not improved, and the doctors decided we needed to travel to the Neonatal Intensive Care Unit (NICU) via air ambulance for more extensive care. The NICU was located in a regional city, approximately 90 miles away.

The time in the NICU was difficult. The medical staff were concerned about Ethan's blood sugar levels. Since he had minimal body fat, they fluctuated significantly. He had an IV in his stomach, a central line through which the nurses fed him lipids and sugar. His tiny feet looked like raw hamburger, because they were pricked every hour to test his blood sugar levels. Ethan had a feeding tube through his nose where he received breastmilk fortified with high-calorie formula. Furthermore, my ability to be with him was dictated by medical staff who often had conflicting ideas of whether I could hold him, nurse him, had to keep him in his incubator, or could even be present at all.

I share this truncated version of my son's birth not out of self-absorption but to position myself in this research. Like the women I feature in this book, I, too, experienced a difficult childbirth. As a result, I deeply empathize with the women whose stories I tell. This experience and my training as a sociologist fostered a desire to better understand birth trauma. I teamed up with two research assistants, Leanna Keleher and Sarah Deming, who helped me conduct interviews with women who self-identified as having traumatic birth experiences. Though I share my familiarity here in the introduction, the book will not feature my story. Instead, *No Perfect Birth* is about the experiences of the women we interviewed and the broader social forces that cause or exacerbate trauma among mothers with difficult childbirth.

I am certainly not the first person to study trauma during childbirth. There is a breadth of high-quality work on this subject worth introducing. What I do here is different. I provide an analysis of the cultural and structural forces at play in producing and exacerbating mothers' trauma, using women's voices in my analysis.

A BRIEF INTRODUCTION TO SCHOLARSHIP
ON TRAUMATIC BIRTHS

To understand the experiences of the women in our sample, one must first have a sense of the causes and frequency of traumatic birth experiences. In truth, trauma is a variable and difficult topic to analyze; what causes trauma for one woman might not bother another at all. Yet certain events tend to be associated with increased traumatization for mothers, including unplanned cesareans, NICU stays, transfers, health complications for mother and baby, and poor interactions with medical staff. There are also certain conditions, such as a history of psychological challenges, including anxiety, that magnify the experience of trauma in women.[2] Finally, there are issues of access. Postnatal trauma is more likely to emerge in women who lack adequate health coverage and who receive inadequate postnatal care.[3] Confounding all of these factors are the goals women have for childbirth: women who have visions of childbirth that differ greatly from their experience are more likely to experience trauma.[4] Among the women we interviewed, those particularly wounded were often women who desired a home birth with minimal interventions but ended up with a hospital birth, medication, and/or a cesarean.

Because of the imprecise nature of defining traumatic childbirth, it is difficult to estimate how frequently it happens. Further complicating such a count is the fact that trauma survivors in general underreport their conditions. United States culture, too, discourages mothers from talking about or viewing childbirth as anything less than perfect. Scholars estimate that up to 40 percent of pregnant women and 43 percent of mothers within the first fourteen months postpartum struggle with birth-related posttraumatic stress disorder.[5] The average rate of occurrence of postnatal posttraumatic stress disorder is estimated at 4 percent.[6]

A mother's experience of childbirth is complicated and dependent on the interaction and confluence of a number of factors. In fact, women can and do perceive their child's birth as traumatic even if medical providers see it as free from complications.[7] This in part reflects a disconnect that can often occur between doctors and patients. Sorensen and Tschetter argue that a woman's sense of their experience with childbirth is based on their individual perception of the interactions of multiple elements of the birth experience.[8] Factors that may contribute to a mother experiencing childbirth as traumatic while remaining unseen to providers include perceptions of personal failure in childbirth, loss of personal control, and deviation from cultural expectations regarding childbirth.[9]

Low-quality interactions with medical staff are central to a mother's perception of her childbirth as traumatic.[10] Using survey data, Sorenson and Tschetter created a measure of such interactions, called the QPI, or Quality of the Provider Interactions.[11] This measure included actions of, and verbal responses by, medical practitioners in response to a patient's requests. Sorenson and Tschetter concluded that the lower the QPI, the more likely a woman was to experience a traumatic birth. These findings were supported by Harris and Ayers who, employing a questionnaire, found that interpersonal experiences with staff—especially situations in which a mother feels dismissed, ignored, or abandoned—were particularly important in the manifestation of trauma.[12]

Even among births considered, "normal" by medical organizations (i.e., full-term vaginal births with no complications) negative experiences with medical staff can cause mothers to experience symptoms of posttraumatic stress disorder.[13] Psychologists Jo Czarnocka and Pauline Slade gave women, considered to have typical childbirths, questionnaires regarding their experience in the days following childbirth and again six months postpartum. Over 25 percent of participants in their study experienced symptoms of trauma. The authors were able to correlate distinct social and psychological factors with the manifestation of trauma and, among other findings, they concluded that women who experienced multiple symptoms of trauma were more likely to report negative experiences with medical staff. For mothers, childbirth is a significant, life-changing event, but for medical staff, it is routine and common. This disconnect can lead to dissatisfaction or emotional injury to mothers.[14]

Traumatic birth experiences can contribute to both short- and long-term psychological and social problems for mothers. Many women who experienced traumatic births report difficulty in performing tasks related to motherhood such as nursing and bonding or interacting with their children—challenges which can cause developmental and emotional delays for infants.[15] Still others share that experiencing a traumatic childbirth has implications for their relationships and family, such as resultant tensions with their partners and a decrease in the number of children women decide to have.[16] Difficult childbirth can result in women's fear of subsequent pregnancies and births.[17]

While I will explore existing scholarship as it relates to the stories of women we interviewed throughout the book, this brief overview shows that trauma or psychological injury in childbirth is relatively common, the quality of patient–provider interactions plays a central role in a mother's relationship to her child's birth, and distressing childbirths can have lasting, harmful impacts on a mother's relationship to herself, her children, and her partner.

THE PEOPLE AND PLACES FEATURED IN THESE STORIES

To better understand birth trauma, I needed to talk to women who had experienced it. Unfortunately, it was not hard to find participants. Too many women experience difficult or traumatic childbirth. To find mothers who fit this population, I placed notices seeking people who had "difficult or traumatic childbirths" in local Facebook groups aimed to support new mothers. I began talking to women in the summer of 2017. The next fall, I partnered with two students who wanted to help on the project. My research assistants Sarah Deming and Leanna Keleher truly made this project possible. Strong women themselves, they participated in these emotionally devastating interviews, helped with transcription, and added a second (and third) set of eyes for coding the data. They were reliable and skilled.

The women we talked with all had ties to the region of this study: small cities in the rural Inland Northwestern United States. To protect their privacy, and that of the medical teams discussed herein, I use pseudonyms for all people and places mentioned in the text. In this manuscript, I focus primarily on the participants who gave birth to their infants and received care in this region (n=28) to accurately assess the role that context—local structures and cultural narratives—played in the manifestation of traumatic childbirth, but we also interviewed women who had ties to the region but gave birth to their children elsewhere (n=7). There is, however, two instances in which I draw on an interview with a woman outside of the region—in chapter 3 when I discuss Jessica's experience with Medicare and in chapter 7 when I explore Gail's successful interactions with a nurse. I do this because Jessica's experience transcends place and so perfectly illustrates the operation of power in the treatment of women in Medicare in rural communities, while Gail's treatment offers insights into ways obstetric care can be improved.

It is also worth noting that only a few of the women in my sample received a diagnosis of having posttraumatic stress disorder as a result of their births. Because of the aforementioned difficulty in operationalizing and assessing trauma, I chose to use a woman's self-identification of having had a traumatic childbirth to admit participants into our study. Trusting women to share their embodied and experiential knowledge is essential to the performance of accurate science (social or medical) both of which have historically dismissed and ignored women's autonomy and wisdom.[18]

Our interviews with women primarily took place in an old house that had been converted into a nonprofit maternal support center. One of the directors gave us access to the building and her personal office. The space was warm and comfortable. It was also private and had a large supply of tissues, which we all needed. In the event that we could not meet at the maternal support center, we held interviews in private places, including study lounges, women's homes, and private reservable rooms at coffeeshops. Two of the included interviews were conducted over the phone.

The interviews usually lasted longer than an hour, about 80 minutes on average. The shortest interview was 40 minutes and the longest was 120.

Only one researcher attended each interview. Interviews were audio-recorded with participants' permission. We began by simply asking women to tell us their birth story. This typically ended up as the bulk of the interview. Once women were done, we used an interview guide to ask follow-up questions about their experience. We asked about salient moments or events. We also inquired about the type of support women had, the interventions they experienced, how having a difficult birth impacted their values, beliefs, and relationships, and the cultural pressures they experienced. We transcribed the interviews ourselves and assigned pseudonyms to all mothers, infants, and other people mentioned, including doctors, nurses, and other medical staff. We kept pseudonyms for staff consistent across interviews to enhance our analysis. Our full interview guide and a list of participants included in this book, along with basic information about them and their birth, can be found in the Appendix.

While we conducted these interviews, we also developed what social scientists call "codes"—a way of identifying or marking the patterns and themes that emerge using inductive analysis.[19] We coded the data to assess these patterns but also to begin the process of theory building. We stopped interviewing women once the information provided was no longer new—when the patterns, ideas, and themes repeated those used by other participants. In sociological research we call this saturation, defined by sociologist Ryanne Pilgeram as the "point in the process where [the researcher is] no longer learning something new and . . . [is] confident that [they] had effectively learned what there was to know about the questions [they] had posed."[20] To validate our codes after completing the interviews, and reassure ourselves that saturation had been met, we each coded the same five interviews and tested our coding system for reliability using NVivo qualitative analysis software. Once we were certain we all interpreted the codes identically, we divided the remaining interviews for coding. I coded all of the interviews, and Sarah and Leanna each coded half such that two people coded each interview.

Most women in the study live in one of two small cities, similar in size, population, and culture, near one another but in two different states: Idaho and Washington. We chose these locations because of their proximity to the research team and their characteristics as rural communities that rely upon regional hospitals for advanced care. As a result of the state boundary, each town has its own small critical access hospital. Critical access hospitals are located in rural areas to provide emergency services. They have fewer than twenty-five beds and do not offer long-term care.[21] Other women featured here come from nearby rural areas. Each received care at one of the two local critical access hospitals in these cities. The first I call North Hospital, located in Springfield, Idaho. North Hospital also runs a series of local clinics in the urban cluster as well as in local rural communities. The hospital sees around 60,000 people annually including emergency, inpatient, and outpatient services. It is the main medical care provider for the surrounding area in a 50-mile radius. The second I call South Hospital, located in Greenfield, Washington. South Hospital also runs a series of regional clinics and has partnerships with a number of local and rural doctors. They see approximately 13,000 emergency visits, 1,600 inpatient visits (including newly birthed infants), and 82,000 outpatients.

As critical access hospitals, North and South Hospitals are not equipped with advanced care resources. Rather, they partner with an air ambulance and urban hospitals for the transfer of critical cases. Many women in this sample experienced transfers to the NICU in two urban hospitals about 90 miles away. The two urban hospitals are located near one another. They are both run by Catholic organizations.[22] One hosts a Level III NICU which has advanced care for babies born extremely premature, who are very sick, or who need surgeries. The other has a Level IV NICU which has all the services of a Level III NICU and is also designated to provide the most complex levels of care for infants with critical conditions.

Before I turn to an explanation of what can be expected in this book, I would like to make an important note. Not all people who give birth are women. Nor are all people who give birth mothers. Because my sample consists entirely of people who identify as both women and mothers and because English lacks more inclusive terms, I use this language. However, I hope this book will soon be outdated because of the emergence of more accurate language that encompasses the experiences of all people who give birth and raise birth children. It is also worth mentioning that transgender and genderqueer people are likely to experience additional trauma in childbirth, above those covered here.

THIS BOOK'S CONTRIBUTION

I am certainly not the first scholar to suggest the U.S. healthcare system fails its patients or that American cultural norms around health care are short-sighted and have harmful effects on the most vulnerable. There are books, too numerous to count, focused on exactly these topics. These pages reflect my attempt to make this failure personal by connecting it to the experience of women in childbirth. I explore the individual trauma resulting from discursive and structural barriers present in rural healthcare systems. Here, I tell the stories of the women who have survived. I look at how their negative experiences with difficult childbirths are exacerbated by institutional and sociopolitical forces.

As a social scientist, I conduct this analysis through engaging with the ideas and work of others. In 1967, sociologists Barney Glaser and Anseim Strauss published *The Discovery of Grounded Theory: Strategies for Qualitative Research.* This book launched a new era of qualitative social science setting it apart from traditional quantitative models. The authors contend that qualitative research should be considered a method whereby scholars generate new theories rather than testing hypotheses.[23] In other words, in qualitative research, scholars find patterns in the data and develop theories based on the work itself. We then return to the cannon to see what existing theories may match, compliment, or improve our work.[24]

I applied this approach in my analysis and found three elements that repeatedly and consistently emerged as factors contributing to women's experiences of trauma during childbirth: *time*, *space*, and *routine*. I also found that women's experiences of trauma occurred as a result of embedded institutional and cultural norms that were invisible to the people operating within the system (both medical staff and mothers themselves). Once I had my nascent theory developed, I excitedly looked through existing research and found identical themes within the work of French philosopher Michael Foucault whose study of sexuality, the body, state control, and the circulation of knowledge revolutionized the way that social scientists think about state power.

Among other contributions, Foucault coined the concept of "biopower," defined as the "numerous and diverse techniques for achieving the subjugations of bodies and the control of populations."[25] Power functions first via the creation of a system of knowledge and second by people's desire to conform to the values and behavior this knowledge constructs. Systems of knowledge become a collectively taken-for-granted truth that serves as the foundation upon which social structures are built and people operate.[26]

For Foucault, this power is exerted through the various institutions of society and the people who serve within them. Foucault contends that institutions exert power on citizens in subtle ways: it may be the structure of a given *space*, the constraints of *time*, and the embedded *routines*—the very themes that arose in my interviews with mothers. He goes on to demonstrate how institutions enforce their power through heavy surveillance of those who operate within them. To those within a given society, it appears that these constraints are objective and real, obscuring the way some lives are structurally privileged over others.

Perhaps most important is the invisibility of this power's reproduction. Using his concepts of governmentality and discipline, Foucault argues that power is applied not only through direct governance but also through impacting the norms and discourse of a society and, in turn, the very way people feel they ought to think and behave even in the absence of direct orders or coercion. As these discourses are embedded into social systems, they become an invisible, taken-for-granted, system of knowledge. As a result, biopower manifests as "a power bent on generating forces, making them grow, and ordering them, rather than one dedicated to impending them, making them submit or destroying them."[27] In this shadow form, then, social structures and the people acting within such systems continue to reproduce social hierarchies, often through violence. Those engaged with the maintenance of such ideologically encoded violence are often unaware of the discourses within which they operate and, in turn, serve to reproduce. In the case of childbirth, we will see how social knowledge which devalues women, in general, and women of color, in particular, are enacted through the practice of health care and by those who practice medicine.

I use Foucault's concept of biopower to frame my analysis of traumatic birth experience. I lean heavily on his understanding that *time, space,* and *routine* are institutional methods of discipline and that the very knowledge systems that inform institutions are internalized by individuals. The structure of health care, to begin with, places overwhelming pressure on the medical staff. In turn, doctors and nurses suffer from overwork and resultant exhaustion as they treat patients. They are disciplined through their use, and lack, of *time.* This condition of time scarcity places a mental and emotional toll on providers, limits their ability to be present with patients, and simultaneously damages mothers' experiences. As the book continues, I explore how the broader bureaucratic processes of medical care are built upon historical concepts of women's value and, as a result, continue to injure women in their inflexibility and resultant inhumanity. I pay particular attention to the way women are hurt by the *space* and *routines* embedded within the healthcare system and practiced by medical staff.

These structural barriers are supported and enforced by an American culture that views health care as a commodity, rather than a human right, and concurrently devalues women. Medical staff and mothers internalize these values and behave and think in ways that exacerbate women's trauma. The cultural norms about ideal childbirth and motherhood injure women who feel they have fallen short, causing significant postnatal mental health challenges. These traumas have long-term impacts on mothers and their relationships.

My selection of Foucault was not taken lightly. Rather, I am aware of how social science has ignored the voices of marginalized scholars, in general, and women scholars, in particular, to the detriment of both science and participants. While his theory serves as a strong scaffold for my work, I also integrate additional feminist theorists and scholars throughout the chapters, bringing in additional voices, theories, and perspectives.

Finally, it is worth noting that this book does not seek to blame either mothers or healthcare providers for experiences of trauma. This focus is too small to capture the way that power operates within obstetric care and erases their dual positions as both victims of institutional power and heroes that push against it. Rather, as a sociologist, I am interested in how systemic power affects people operating within its sphere. Thus, in this book, I contextualize women's experiences within the U.S. healthcare system and the country's dominant ideologies.

CHAPTER ORGANIZATION

To explore how institutions and ideologies perpetuate mothers' experiences of trauma, I begin each chapter with one participant's story and connect this case to the chapter's themes and relevant social theories. I follow this introduction with a deeper analysis that interweaves mothers' stories with existing scholarship. This enables me to put women's lived experiences in their appropriate context to more accurately show how power operates in obstetric care. It is worth noting that the experiences women share may be distressing to readers.

Chapter 1 explains how the structures of American healthcare create a system in which doctors are not permitted the *time* they need with patients. The private insurance model of care requires efficiency and profit to be central to the healthcare process. To succeed in these goals, doctors are forced to see many patients quickly. This coupled with the severe shortage of medical practitioners results in an impossible system. Doctors are overworked and unable to provide time, presence of mind, and associated high-quality interactions with their patients. This lack of time is injurious to mothers, which I demonstrate using the stories of our participants to highlight the impact of poor-quality interpersonal interactions between patients and medical practitioners on the manifestation of trauma.

In the second chapter, I look more deeply at the way *space* is used to inadvertently harm women in childbirth. Here I examine the historical division between midwifery and hospital obstetric care and how this separation hurts women who needed to transfer between the two. I also look at the creation of the NICU and how the spatial separation of women from their infants causes significant injury to mothers.

The third chapter looks at how bureaucratic practices, or *routines*, and the practices of care hurt mothers. I start by talking about the inflexibility and uncompassionate way bureaucracies function. I further explore how actors within an institution (doctors, nurses, and even patients) are herded through policies and practices (routines or habits) in ways that perpetuate and cause harm. To explain the inhumanity of bureaucracy, I turn to specific examples as they apply to traumatic childbirth and the women in my sample: access to care, treatment while their child is hospitalized, and broader trends regarding infant and maternal mortality.

The fourth chapter uses the example of obstetric violence to extend structural analysis and examine how time, space, routine but also ideology injures women during childbirth. To do this, I investigate the role of historic social hierarchies used to justify the use of state repression and control of women's bodies. These cultural and ideological artifacts remain hidden in the shadows of contemporary culture. Through an examination of obstetric violence, we are able to see how these discursive shadows emerge in ways that devalue women—particularly women of color—and undermine women's power in contemporary obstetric care.

Chapter 5 examines how these discourses (or systems of knowledge) are internalized by women to their detriment. To do this, I provide a brief history of obstetric care in the United States and the evolving norms and values around childbirth. I then show how the belief that so-called "natural" birth is best, held by many women in Springfield and Greenfield, serves to both control women's bodies and create psychological pain when mothers are unable to attain these goals.

In chapter 6, I move beyond the experience of childbirth itself to look at the impact difficult births have on women. Here I build on work regarding the consequence of trauma on a mother's relationship with her children and partner.[28] I do this by both continuing my critique of the discursive harm done to women while also pointing to the structural shortcomings in postpartum care.

Chapter 7 uses the narratives of mothers highlighting successful interactions with medical staff to develop a framework of intervention. I draw upon the ideas presented by the women we interviewed who use power by demanding *time*, *space*, and new *routines* from their providers. The solutions women propose are not farfetched. Rather, I show examples of them by looking at the interventions and models happening in other nations (i.e., "rooming-in" with infants in the neonatal intensive care unit or improving patient–provider communication).[29]

Finally, in the conclusion, I summarize the contributions of this book. I then consider the possibilities for improvement that can be gathered from looking at models of care in other nations. I ultimately expand Foucault's theories using the work of postmodern feminists Susan Bordo, Judith Butler, and Sara Ahmed to consider the potential for change.

NOTES

1. Pseudonyms are used to protect people's privacy throughout this manuscript.

2. Eelco Olde, Onno van der Hart, Rolf Kleber, and Maarten van Son, "Posttraumatic stress following childbirth: A review," *Clinical Psychology Review* 26, no. 1 (2006): 1–16.

3. Madeleine Simpson and Christine Catling, "Understanding psychological traumatic birth experiences: A literature review," *Women and Birth* 29, no. 3 (2016): 203–207.

4. Simpson and Catling, "Understanding psychological traumatic birth experiences," 203–207; Anne Denis, Olivier Parant, and Stacey Callahan, "Post-traumatic stress disorder related to birth: a prospective longitudinal study in a French population," *Journal of Reproductive and Infant Psychology* 29, no. 2 (2011): 125–135.

5. Pelin Dikmen Yildiz, Susan Ayers, and Louise Phillips, "The prevalence of posttraumatic stress disorder in pregnancy and after birth: A systematic review and meta-analysis," *Journal of Affective Disorders* 208 (2017): 634–645.

6. Yildiz et al., "The prevalence of posttraumatic stress disorder," 634–645.

7. Simpson and Catling, "Understanding psychological traumatic birth experiences," 203–207.

8. Dianna Spies Sorenson and Lois Tschetter, "Prevalence of negative birth perception, disaffirmation, perinatal trauma symptoms, and depression among postpartum women," *Perspectives in Psychiatric Care* 46, no. 1 (2010): 14–25.

9. Simpson and Catling, "Understanding psychological traumatic birth experiences," 203–207.

10. Simpson and Catling, "Understanding psychological traumatic birth experiences," 203–207.

11. Sorenson and Tschetter, "Prevalence of negative birth perception," 14–25.

12. Rachel Harris and Susan Ayers, "What makes labour and birth traumatic? A survey of intrapartum 'hotspots'," *Psychology & Health* 27, no. 10 (2012): 1166–1177.

13. Jo Czarnocka and Pauline Slade, "Prevalence and predictors of post-traumatic stress symptoms following childbirth," *British Journal of Clinical Psychology* 39, no. 1 (2000): 35–51; Simpson and Catling, "Understanding psychological traumatic birth experiences," 203–207; World Health Organization, "Care in normal birth: A practical guide," *Birth* 24, no. 2 (1997).

14. Christiana Macdougall, "'Oh, Get Over It. I Do This Every Day': How ignoring the specialness of childbirth contributes to experiences of emotional distress," *Journal of the Motherhood Initiative for Research and Community Involvement* 9, no. 2 (2018).

15. Cheryl Beck and Sue Watson, "Impact of birth trauma on breast-feeding: A tale of two pathways," *Nursing Research* 57, no. 4 (2008): 228–236; John Davies, Pauline Slade, Ingram Wright, and Peter Stewart, "Posttraumatic stress symptoms following childbirth and mothers' perceptions of their infants," *Infant Mental Health Journal: Official Publication of The World Association for Infant Mental Health* 29, no. 6 (2008): 537–554; Simpson and Catling, "Understanding psychological traumatic birth experiences," 203–207.

16. Susan Ayers, Daniel B. Wright, and Nicola Wells, "Symptoms of post-traumatic stress disorder in couples after birth: Association with the couple's relationship and parent–baby bond," *Journal of Reproductive and Infant Psychology* 25, no. 1 (2007): 40–50; Karin Gottvall and Ulla Waldenström, "Does a traumatic birth experience have an impact on future reproduction?," *BJOG: An International Journal of Obstetrics and Gynaecology* 109, no. 3 (2002): 254–260.

17. Christina Nilsson, Eva Robertson, and Ingela Lundgren, "An effort to make all the pieces come together: Women's long-term perspectives on their experiences of intense fear of childbirth," *International Journal of Childbirth* 2, no. 4 (2012): 255–268.

18. Camille Pagán, "When Doctors Downplay Women's Health Concerns," *New York Times.* May 3, 2018, https://www.nytimes.com/2018/05/03/well/live/when-doctors-downplay-womens-health-concerns.html; Gabrielle Levy, "Dying to be Heard," *US News and World Report.* April 20, 2018, https://www.usnews.com/news/the-report/articles/2018-04-20/why-women-struggle-to-get-doctors-to-believe-them; Joan Always, "The trouble with gender: Tales of the still-missing feminist revolution in social theory," *Sociological Theory* 13, no. 3 (1995): 209–228.

19. Sarah Luker, *Salsa Dancing in the Social Sciences: Research in an Age of Info-Glut* (Cambridge, MA: Harvard University Press, 2008).

20. Ryanne Pilgeram. *Pushed Out: Contested Development and Rural Gentrification in the US West* (Seattle, WA: University of Washington Press, 2021).

21. "Critical Access Hospitals," Rural Health Information Hub, accessed November 17, 2020, https://www.ruralhealthinfo.org/topics/critical-access-hospitals.

22. Approximately 17% of all hospitals in the United States are part of the Catholic healthcare system. In many regions, they are the only provider available to residents (Katie Hafner, "As Catholic Hospitals expand, so do limits on some procedures," *The New York Times.* August 10, 2018. https://www.nytimes.com/2018/08/10/health/catholic-hospitals-procedures.html).

23. Barney Glaser and Anselm Strauss, *The Discovery of Grounded Theory* (New York: Routledge, 2017); Luker, *Salsa Dancing*; Charles Ragan, *The Comparative Method: Moving Beyond Qualitative and Quantitative Strategies* (Berkeley, CA: University of California Press, 1987).

24. Brené Brown, *Dare to Lead* (New York: Random House, 2018).

25. Michel Foucault, *The History of Sexuality*, vol. 1 (New York: Vintage, 1998).

26. Michel Foucault, *Society Must be Defended: Lectures at the College de France 1975–1976* (New York: Picador Press, 2003).

27. Foucault, *The History of Sexuality.*

28. Beck and Watson, "Impact of birth trauma on breast-feeding," 228–236; Davies, Slade, Wright, and Stewart, "Posttraumatic stress symptoms following childbirth," 537–554.

29. Francisco De Carvalho Guerra Abecasis and Antonio Gomes, "Rooming-in for preterm infants: How far should we go? Five-year experience at a tertiary hospital," *Acta Paediatrica* 95, no. 12 (2006): 1567–1570; Shimon Weiss, Eric Goldlust, and Yvonne Vaucher, "Improving parent satisfaction: An intervention to increase neonatal parent-provider communication," *Journal of Perinatology* 30, no. 6 (2010): 425–430.

Chapter 1

"The Most Horrible Part"

The Trauma Imposed by Time

Ashley was thirty weeks pregnant when she began to sense something was wrong. Frightened, she called her doctor and reported that she was unable to eat, felt extremely nauseous, and her hands and face were swollen. Her doctor dismissed her concerns saying, "It's just the end of pregnancy. It's normal." Ashley felt frustrated, intuitively knowing that it was not normal for her to be unable to muster the energy to leave her home, much less her bed.

At her thirty-six-week appointment, Ashley's fears proved justified when her doctors measured her blood pressure at 200/150. Optimal blood pressure in adults is 120/80. Elevated blood pressure in pregnancy can indicate several troubling situations including preeclampsia, a condition of pregnancy characterized by high blood pressure, protein in a mother's urine, and swollen limbs.[1] Left untreated, preeclampsia can develop into eclampsia, the onset of seizures and, potentially, organ failure. Ashley's doctor immediately sent her to the hospital and started her on magnesium sulfate.[2]

Commonly known as Epsom Salt, magnesium sulfate is a mineral used internally to prevent seizures in pregnant women experiencing preeclampsia, offer neural protections for premature infants, and delay childbirth.[3] The internal use of magnesium sulfate leaves people feeling tired, nauseous, dizzy, and generally unwell, among other potential, and more severe, side effects. Preeclampsia arises in approximately 2–8 percent of childbirths globally and approximately 63,000 people die annually from preeclampsia or eclampsia.[4]

Despite the intervention, Ashley's blood pressure continued to rise. She felt like she was "just fading away" and her doctors feared she would experience a seizure or stroke, possible outcomes of preeclampsia. They decided she needed to have an emergency cesarean. Birth of the child is the only way to reliably end preeclampsia and its symptoms.[5]

Like many of the women in our sample, Ashley does not recall all the events that occurred between being notified of the need for an emergency cesarean and the birth of her child. Memory loss is a common outcome of the experience of trauma.[6] Yet, she does remember the feeling of panic as they rushed her on a gurney through the hospital to the operating room. She recollects "the fluorescent lighting passing over" and people rushing around.

Once in the operating room, Ashley was strapped down to the operating table—a practice still performed at some, but not all, hospitals. Reflecting on the event, Ashley recalls, "It is such a creepy feeling. The lights are so bright. I remember being so ashamed because I was not expecting this to happen." Ashley's shame deepened when her doctor informed her that he would be shaving her pubic hair. "I had the full bush going on and then some. It just made me feel so exposed and embarrassed and there's all these lights and all these people around and they're shaving me. It just felt gross."

Beyond feelings of embarrassment, Ashley felt "terrified . . . It's very violent, the c-section. You're moving around on the table, really. Your body, they're tugging and pulling. I remember I had tears streaming down my face." When her daughter was finally born, Ashley was able to see her for only a moment before the medical team "whisked her away to go into a warmer."

After her daughter was removed from the room, Ashley's doctor said "Okay, Ashley, I'm gonna sew up these abs of yours." This comment felt unsettling and inappropriately informal to Ashley, who thought, "Why the fuck would you say something like that?" Ashley was then taken to the intensive care unit where she was left alone, with no feeling in her lower body, for approximately ninety minutes. She believed that she had no way of calling a nurse and no knowledge of the status of her infant. She remembers the experience as "scary because I could not move, and I had no idea what was going on."

Finally, Ashley was taken to the maternity ward, where she was placed on a catheter and IV (on which hurried staff repeatedly became entangled) and was finally able to see her daughter. She felt incredibly "detached" from her infant, "when she was born, I remember not wanting to see her, which made me feel horrible." Ashley stayed in the hospital for ten days because her blood pressure remained high, even after giving birth to her daughter. During this time, her baby was also unwell. She was lethargic and struggling from the magnesium sulfate that entered her body while she was still in Ashley's uterus. Hypotonia—low muscle tone and strength—is a common side effect of magnesium sulfate in infants.[7] As she finally left the hospital, Ashley continued to hear her doctor's parting words in her mind: "We're really happy you're here because we did not think you were going to be."

Ashley's experience was objectively traumatic. She nearly died. Yet, it is also clear that her experience of trauma was intensified by certain interactions—or a lack of interactions—on the part of hospital staff. Her doctor failed to *take time* to listen to her concerns and investigate the symptoms she reported. In their rush to perform the cesarean, they failed to adequately administer her anesthesia. She was not given time with her daughter following the surgery, and subsequently struggled to form a bond with her baby. Other factors that contributed to the poor interactions between Ashley and her doctor are more subtle in their reflection of time. Her doctor used crass language discussing her body, which made her feel dehumanized. Had he taken time to consider his words and their impact and to interact from a place of compassion and mindfulness, these episodes may have been prevented. Such clarity of mind requires doctors to have time themselves, time to process events and reflect. As this chapter explores, the structures of U.S. rural obstetric care fail to afford medical practitioners the time they need to interact positively with patients.

As discussed in the introductory chapter, social scientists have documented how negative interactions with medical providers significantly impact a mother's likelihood of experiencing trauma following childbirth. What needs better conceptualization are the factors that cause poor quality interactions between patients and providers. It is here, where theory can help. According to Foucault, power operates in all interactions; it is a tool (not a position) that can be used by all people.[8] Philosopher Susan Bordo furthers Foucault's theory in her work "Feminism, Foucault, and the Body" arguing that even though no one person has or controls power, power impacts people differently depending on their social position.[9] In the context of medical care, we see that people in certain positions (doctors) have more possibility to use power than others (patients).

In this chapter, I explore how institutional and ideological constraints on *time* result in poor interactions between patients and providers. Using Foucault's method of genealogy—the analytical practice of tracing the "constitution of knowledges, discourses, domains of objects, and so on."[10]—to examine how discourse and power/knowledge developed. As a result, we are better able to witness how taken-for-granted truths of a society are simply the product of a particular historical trajectory and not objectively true or right. It is with this practice in mind that one can evaluate the creation of the U.S. healthcare system and its unique reliance on employer-based private insurance. To do so, I first explain the institutional operation of time through tracing the history of the U.S. insurance-based healthcare system. I then focus on one particular weakness of this system that significantly manages time, massive staffing shortages. In considering the impact of a lack of doctors, I focus particularly on rural obstetric care (given that the women I interviewed reside in rural communities and are impacted by its stark scarcity) and the way that time, specifically a lack of time, is used to control doctors. Finally, I present examples from our participant's stories of poor patient-provider interactions to establish how the constraints of a doctor's time impacts the quality of care.

TIME

In Foucault's work on biopower, he argues that systems of knowledge are built into the structures of society and both govern and discipline human bodies and reproduction. These structures control the time, space, and routine of the people within their sphere in ways that reinforce and reproduce this knowledge and create, in his words, "docile bodies."[11] This knowledge is further internalized by people as norms and values such that they behave in ways they feel they should even without direct orders or coercion.

In this chapter, I consider the operation of time specifically. In *Discipline and Punishment,* Foucault argues that through the control of time, institutions "establish rhythms, impose particular occupations, regulate the cycles of repetition."[12] It is through the use and management of time that institutions create discipline among those who operate within them. Consider for example, a visit to the doctor's office. Internalizing the time structures in the institution, a patient arrives and immediately knows what to do (routines organized in time) without direct order or coercion. They check in at the front desk. Sit in the waiting area. Follow the nurse when their name is called. Behavior is controlled through these internalized, temporal expectations.

Foucault does not distinguish between knowledge and power. They are, rather, one in the same, "power/knowledge." Power is produced via collectively accepted knowledge, scientific claims, and perceived "truth." Truth, to Foucault, is constructed by societies through the production and acceptance of discourses. In turn, power "produces; it produces reality; it produces domains of objects and rituals of truth."[13]

A BRIEF GENEALOGY OF U.S. HEALTH CARE

The first movement toward government-run health care in the United States was in the creation of the U.S. Marine Hospital Service in 1798. This program was funded through a salary deduction for members, paving the way for the practice of connecting medical care to one's employment. The U.S. Marine Hospital Service served as the foundation for what became the U.S. Public Health Service in 1912, following a series of name changes.[14] Today the Public Health Service oversees several divisions within the broader Department of Health and Human Services including the National Institutes of Health (NIH), the Centers for Disease Control and Prevention (CDC),

Indian Health Service (IHS), Food and Drug Administration (FDA), and several lesser-known agencies.[15]

As with other political conflicts at the time, the conversation around health care reflected tension between deeply held beliefs of U.S. society. These debates featured a strong ideological split between those who advocated for a strong federalized system, led by Alexander Hamilton, and those who advocated for the states' rights to dictate such programs, steered by Thomas Jefferson.[16] While the uniquely U.S. fear of centralized control over health care ultimately prevails, even Jefferson was swayed to support some national healthcare initiatives when he learned of a bill in Congress aimed to make cowpox vaccines free and available to the public.[17]

Concurrent to these debates was the evolution of the hospital system. Until the mid-1800s, hospitals largely served to shelter people who were of low income or those who had contagious illnesses.[18] Medical professionals had little ability to heal or even prevent illnesses until medical advances at the beginning of the twentieth century.[19]

Following the Civil War, federal health care evolved in response to a yellow fever outbreak in 1878. Again, debate ensued between southern states that rejected healthcare programs at the federal level and northern states that advocated for the creation of a National Board of Health. The Board was ultimately formed in 1879, yet it met strong opposition from states who perceived federal involvement in health care as governmental overreach.[20]

As medical advancements were made in the ability of physicians to diagnose and care for people with contagious diseases, hospitals began to increase in cost. Yet, more significant to many people in the United States were the expenses they accrued with absence from work.[21] Fraternal organizations, other benevolent societies, and labor unions in the United States sought to protect income for employees but focused little on the actual cost of health care.[22] Even the first national "sick benefit program," founded by the Granite Cutters Union in 1877, focused on income lost as opposed to coverage of health expenses.[23]

Over the next several decades, employers began to provide care for on-the-job injuries and broader medical benefits for employees and others in the community.[24] Doctors resisted these programs, because they viewed them as a threat to their professional autonomy and earnings. Workers were also unsatisfied, as the model resulted in doctors who were loyal to the company, rather than the patient, and often failed to have their patient's best interests in mind.[25]

Finally, in 1910, the Progressive Party, led by President Theodore Roosevelt, made it a priority to fight for universal health insurance and included the creation of national health insurance in its 1912 election platform.[26] This battle was ultimately lost in response to the growing conservative movement at the end of World War I and the overt resistance of the American Medical Association (AMA) to universal health care.[27]

For the next twenty years, the federal government engaged very little with the discussion of health care, except for veterans.[28] However, the Great Depression led to a significant shift in thinking regarding poverty and government welfare services with an increase in support for social welfare policies and programs.[29] Yet, even during this period of support for social services, health care was dropped from the Social Security Law of 1935 for fear the entire bill would fail to pass.[30]

Instead, what was then called prepaid group health care—and ultimately became health maintenance organizations (HMOs) under President Nixon—began in earnest. The first such program, Blue Cross, was created in Texas in the 1930s and was supported by large, often wealthy organized healthcare systems, such as hospitals.[31] These HMO programs swiftly evolved and often varied from one another. Many programs that featured greater levels of consumer control and physician choice were opposed by the AMA and medical providers.[32]

By 1960, there were 700 insurance companies in the United States. As prepaid group health care increased so too did the problems that continue to plague American health care today, staffing shortages and cost-prohibitive care.[33] Throughout these decades, the AMA continued to oppose federal healthcare initiatives and instead advanced the states' rights narratives regarding the provision of health care.[34] The U.S. obsession with limited federal government has ironically led to the excessive power and dominance of massive private corporations over citizen's health.[35]

The legislation creating Medicare and Medicaid was passed in 1962 under the Kennedy administration. These programs provide federally orchestrated federal healthcare benefits for people who were retired or had a disability (Medicare) and those who were low-income (Medicaid). Since then, work requirements have been placed on Medicaid eligibility (Personal Responsibility and Work Opportunities Act of 1996). Under the Affordable Care Act, many states elected to expand the financial boundaries for qualification of Medicaid. In Idaho and Washington, where this study took place, this allowed an additional 53,000 people and 644,000 people, respectively, to access the Medicaid system.

Beyond Medicaid, the 1990s and 2000s saw healthcare costs in the United States continue to skyrocket.[36] Today, the U.S. Health Care system is the most expensive in the world. The per capita expense in the United States is approximately $9,892 as compared with a median rate for members of the Organization for Economic Cooperation and Development (OECD) of $4,033. People in the United States pay more for medication, see higher costs associated with medical services, are dependent on employment for coverage, face high deductibles and copays, and pay greater prices for hospital adminis-tration.[37] In 2018, there were nearly 250,000 GoFundMe campaigns in which people sought to raise money for medical care.[38] Over half a million families in the United States file bankruptcy every year as a result of overwhelming medical bills, often despite having insurance.[39]

Notwithstanding the exorbitant costs, the relative quality of U.S. health care is rapidly decreasing. Between 1990 and 2016, the United States dropped from sixth to twenty-seventh in health status ranking according to the Global Burden of Diseases, Injuries, and Risk Factors Study.[40] This decline in rank reflects both the lack of investment in health care by the U.S. federal government over the past thirty years (proportionate to sky-rocketing costs) as well as an improvement in health outcomes for residents of countries that have universal health coverage. While this study shows a global drop in U.S. ranking, the United States has consistently performed below other wealthy nations in terms of health outcomes.[41] U.S. health care, in general, and maternal care, in particular, rank beneath similar nations in terms of healthcare access, speed, and equality of care while also costing far more.[42]

The U.S. health system is perhaps the best example of what anthropologist Elizabeth Hsu views as the undermining of medical professionalism.[43] Under the ideological guise of individualism, freedom, and personal control, the United States placed its healthcare system in the hands of private companies whose goals are not the improvement of public health but the fattening of their executive's wallets.

The move to employer-based, private insurance was not accidental. Rather, it reflects key systems of knowledge reinforced at crucial moments in his-tory: the connection of insurance to employment with the creation of the U.S. Marine Hospital System and employer-provided healthcare facilities. As HMOs expanded, because of demand, so too did the goal of health care change from a focus on patient health to the creation of profit.[44] The search for profit drives the costs for healthcare treatments up while attempting to keep expenses for insurers and hospitals low. As a result of this profit-driven incentivization, the system remains plagued with severe staffing shortages restricting doctor's *time*, among other disastrous problems.

RURAL HEALTH CARE

Within the United States, the problems associated with employer- and insurance-based health care are not distributed equally, they dispropor-tionately affect rural areas. This is not accidental. Managed care efforts to reduce healthcare costs and improve quality of care have neglected rural communities.[45] Here, then, I turn my focus to rural health care and explore how the problems outlined above impact residents.

The U.S. Census defines rural based on its relationship to, or as the antithesis of, urban. According to their website, rural is "any population, housing, or territory NOT in an urban area."[46] Urban areas are defined as those which have 50,000 or more residents, while "urban clusters," concentrated residences outside of urban areas, have between 2,500 and 50,000 inhabitants. Approximately 19 percent of the U.S. population, about 60 million people, lived in rural areas at the time of the 2010 Census. This number has consistently decreased, so it is safe to predict these numbers will be lower in the 2020 Census.

Rural communities are plagued by a lack of jobs and high poverty rates. While not new challenges, as opportunities in farming, mining, and manufacturing have ebbed in recent years, this problem has grown. The economic vitality of rural areas is often reliant upon a single industry (e.g., a mine, a factory, farming) so as these opportunities leave, there are few alternatives for residents.[47] At the same time, rural areas often see a "brain drain" wherein the people who can access high levels of education leave for urban areas with more opportunity. Such high rates of unemployment and poverty result in a patient population that is disproportionately likely to be uninsured or underinsured and at higher risk for chronic illnesses.[48]

The divide between suburban and rural health care is stark. Nineteen percent of U.S. residents live in rural areas, yet only 9 percent of doctors practice in rural communities.[49] State funding cuts over the past twenty years have led to significant hospital closures in rural areas.[50] Rural communities and urban clusters are also more likely to be serviced by what are called Critical Access Hospitals (CAHs). CAHs are hospitals characterized as having 24-hour emergency services, fewer than twenty-five beds, and discharging patients in less than ninety-six hours. These hospitals are also exempt from quality standards as outlined in the 2010 Affordable Care Act.[51]

While U.S. hospitals in general are struggling with staffing shortages due to funding shortfalls, this is particularly true for hospitals and medical care centers in rural communities.[52] Of the 7,200 areas in the United States designated by the Health Resources and Services Administration as "Health Professional Shortage Areas," 60 percent are in rural areas.[53] The Association of American Medical Colleges (AAMC) estimates that by 2032 the shortfall of physicians will rise to 122,000—meaning the United States will require the services of 122,000 more physicians than will be practicing.[54] They expect this demand to be felt throughout the United States but most predominantly in urban and rural centers. The doctors that do practice in rural communities are often generalists who can work in a variety of areas.

Therefore, an additional shortage of specialists also exists in rural communities. Medical practitioners who choose to work in rural areas are typically paid in ways equivalent to their urban peers, but often work longer hours and have fewer resources.[55]

Despite their greater need for care, people living in rural communities often lack access to medical services. Turning to obstetric care in particular, rural women are more likely to have high-risk pregnancies and babies are disproportionately in need of advanced postnatal care. Yet, women considered to be "high risk" and living in rural areas are less frequently referred to a fully equipped hospital than are women in nonrural areas.[56] These same regions often lack access to neonatal intensive care units (NICUs) and even basic services, such as hospitals and maternal health care. As a result, people have to travel further distances for emergency or inpatient healthcare services or, in the case of childbirth, rely on out-of-hospital birth services such as home births or even forego prenatal care altogether.[57] Further complicating the issue is the fact that many remaining hospitals are affiliated with the Catholic church, such as the two urban hospitals the women in our study transferred to for more extensive care, and therefore may not provide important reproductive health services such as emergency contraception, reproductive support services for infertility, emergency care for pregnancy complications, or some testing and support for sexually transmitted diseases due to directives under which they operate.[58]

Nationally, obstetricians work approximately forty to sixty hours per week in addition to their nights on-call in which they respond to urgent or emergency situations.[59] According to a Medscape survey of 20,000 medical professionals, obstetricians report long work hours as the second most challenging part of their job (behind the volume of rules and regulations).[60] There is a severe shortage of obstetricians and gynecologists; the American Congress of Obstetricians and Gynecologists estimates a shortage of "6,000 to 8,000 OB-GYNs by 2020." There are currently 20,000 OB-GYNs and 12,000 nurse-midwives practicing medicine.

As with the broader physical shortage, rural communities bear the brunt of the nation's lack of obstetricians. Half of the counties (mostly rural) in the United States do not have an obstetrician-gynecologist while 56 percent do not have a nurse midwife.[61] In fact, only 20 percent of rural counties have obstetric care.[62] In Idaho, where most of the women we interviewed live, there are only 152 obstetricians for the state's 784,000 female-bodied residents.[63] Instead, patients depend on midwives, general practitioners, or must travel long distances to access care. While this may be appropriate for a typical birth scenario, it can be incredibly dangerous for women with high-risk pregnancies or surprise complications.

HOW A LACK OF TIME HURTS PATIENT-
PROVIDER INTERACTIONS

Staffing shortages in rural obstetric care have profound impacts on the experiences of patients, particularly women facing difficult birth. Staff shortages often result in more patients per doctor and less time for each patient. Medical staff are not superhuman, though we often expect them to be. The ability of doctors and nurses to be mindful and present with patients is shaped by the structures in which they operate. Staffing shortages and resultant lack of time inevitably put stress on medical staff and affects patient-provider interactions.

As doctors rush to fit in their full load of clients, women often feel unheard or unimportant. These exchanges are restricted and patterned by time. One example comes from our participant Erica who explained the feelings of unimportance felt by many women in our sample by juxtaposing her hospital experience against that which she had with a midwife. She said,

> I don't feel like the doctors are as available as I wish they were, and I don't feel like they care about me as much as my midwife did. I felt like the midwife understood . . . it was an hour-long appointment every time. I'm in and out in twenty minutes with the doctor. I always felt like I was wasting their time when I had questions. I always feel like I have to hurry up 'cause I know that they're waiting for the next patient.

Nearly every woman in our sample who had a hospital birth mentioned the lack of time they had with their doctor as a struggle exacerbating their difficult childbirths.

It is also probable that overworked obstetricians will make decisions that are not ideal for their patients to save time. According to Dr. Marty Makary, evaluation of healthcare systems assesses the process of such things as surgeries but not the rate at which unneeded interventions are performed. He argues that some doctors may face pressures that lead them to perform certain unnecessary and detrimental treatments.[64] One example is the increasingly common cesarean. The cesarean is a serious surgery with significant side effects for women. Though credited with reducing both maternal and infant mortality rates, the overuse of cesarean (discussed further in chapter 5) has significant negative impacts on mothers. Its use in situations in which it is not medically warranted, especially when it is more convenient for a doctor, is particularly disturbing.[65]

Overburdened doctors and medical systems can also lead to long wait times for women who need gynecological care. In the area of this study, it is not unusual for nonpregnant women to wait three or more months for an appointment. Inability to make timely appointments or receive care at all is also a profound barrier for women after they have given birth to their children. Many women reported having severe symptoms of posttraumatic stress disorder or postpartum depression but being unable to access care for their disorders.

With this context in mind, I turn to our data to demonstrate how doctor's lack of time results in low-quality interactions with patients, which causes or exacerbates their experiences of trauma. I focus on three types of interactions: situations in which medical staff fail to effectively communicate with mothers, dismiss women's experiences, and are disrespectful to mothers in their communication. I connect each of these themes to staff's lack of time.[66]

The Traumatizing Experience of Absent Communication

Alice always knew she wanted what is commonly referred to as a "natural childbirth." Thus, when she was pregnant, she decided to give birth in her own home with the support of a local doula and midwife. After twelve hours of labor, she became dehydrated from vomiting and lost strength. Her cervix stopped dilating and it seemed her progress was halting.

Despite her objections, Alice ultimately followed her midwife's recommendation and went to the local hospital to finish her labor with the support of medical tools and interventions. After an additional twelve hours of labor in the hospital, Alice was wheeled down the hall on a gurney to the operating room—in her words—"in hysterics" and ultimately gave birth to her infant. Alice recalls hearing her newborn baby crying and the experience of being separated from her daughter "the most horrible part" of her birth experience. Finally, they brought Elizabeth to meet her mother and then, after a few minutes, sent her to the nursery with her father.

After Alice left the recovery room, the family was reunited in a hospital room in the birth ward. At some point, Alice fell asleep but, when she woke up, Elizabeth was no longer in the room. Alice panicked, "Where's my baby!" She sat there, unable to find her call button and unable to get up, overwhelmed with fear. After what felt like hours but, she acknowledges, was likely a shorter period of time, a nurse entered the room and Alice learned that the staff decided to give Elizabeth an IV but were having difficulty finding a vein. A supporter of attachment parenting—a philosophy that emphasizes parent-child connection through empathy, responsiveness, and physical connection—Alice was irate, "That's the last thing I wanted was for my baby to be somewhere else for two hours getting poked by needles!"[67] Alice slept only in fits and starts for the next two days in the hospital, fearful that the staff would once again take Elizabeth.

This was a common story for women we interviewed. The perceived theft of women's babies, resulting from staff's failure to take the time needed to clearly communicate with patients. As a consequence, women experience heightened anxiety throughout their stay in the hospital that exacerbate the trauma of difficult births. For Alice and others in our sample, a failure to take time results in a loss of trust and a fear of their baby being removed from their room, which exacerbated their anxiety following scary and traumatic births.

In addition to fearing for their child's life, women also felt traumatized by not knowing if they, themselves, would survive. Rhonda recalls the experience of having no information about her own survival:

> The doctor came in at the 45-minute mark and the radiology tech is like stone—won't tell you a damn thing. The doctor came in and said they were going to do a c-section and that was it. He didn't explain anything, he didn't give me any of the results, and as my husband says, it's like all of the nurses popped out of the floor, and things started moving . . . He never told me anything about what was going on, which made me really anxious 'cause now we're in like super-stress mode and I have no idea why . . . I just got more and more anxious. Then they wheeled me into the operating room, and I was breathing pretty hard, I was crying pretty hard . . . I'm not afraid of tears, but I think the doctor was, because it just sort of made him stonewall about giving me anything else. So, I had less information and less access and less anything. And felt pretty . . . . probably one of the most disempowering experiences of my life.

Rhonda's experience with her doctor's care was clearly damaging. He failed to take time to communicate with her about her health and birth. He did things *to* her and explained very little. When he saw her emotional response, he shut down and further withheld information. In his rush, her doctor failed to treat her like a human being in what was an incredibly important moment.

Alice and Rhonda share examples of the pain that new mothers can experience when medical staff fail to take time needed to clearly communicate with patients. While the doctors and nurses unlikely intended to cause harm in these scenarios, they result in acute anxiety for mothers. In Alice's case, nursing staff took her baby because they saw it as the right thing to do— knowledge systems dictated that this was an appropriate norm to follow and failed to take time to share their decision with her. For Rhonda, the control of time deepened her experience of trauma. It is likely that medical staff never thought twice about any of these actions. Rather, they simply followed the scripts established by the broader system of knowledge. They did what was normal, routine. Thus, while this chapter focuses on time, it is clear that institutional power operates through all of these forces in its impact on obstetric care.

The Traumatizing Influence of Dismissed Concerns

It is clear from these stories that medical staff failing to take the time needed for clear communication, especially when it concerns the wellbeing of one's child or oneself, can be particularly traumatic for mothers. A second pattern evident in mothers' stories is how women found that their desires or concerns regarding certain medical procedures were dismissed by doctors.

Meghan's water broke thirty-seven weeks into her pregnancy. Her family immediately brought her to the emergency room at the local critical access hospital where she proceeded to wait an hour to be moved to the labor and delivery unit. After several hours of labor, Meghan's obstetrician recommended a cesarean, because the baby was in distress. Meghan was wheeled to the operating room, but her medical staff was unaware of her latex allergy, so they had to prepare a second room, and she was relocated. The nursing staff then transferred her to the operating bed. However, during the transfer, they "kinked" Meghan's epidural and she "felt this shooting pain go through [her] back." Meghan attempted to notify the staff, but the anesthesiologist discounted her concerns telling her she was "overreacting." Meghan protested saying "No, like, my, my back literally feels like someone is shoving lightning rods into it." Again, the anesthesiologist dismissed her, saying "You're fine. You're just overreacting." Meghan persisted to which the anesthesiologist replied, "I've maxed you out on drugs. There's nothing I can do." But Meghan could "feel them sewing me back together." Again, the anesthesiologist still ignored her concerns, saying, "You're fine . . . It's all in your head. You just think that that's what it is." Meghan proved her wrong by explaining the exact detail of what the doctor and medical team was doing.

Meghan's story was surprisingly common in our sample, with several women reporting that they could feel pain when they were supposed to be anesthetized for their cesarean. While epidurals do not numb a woman's body completely and women can still feel pressure from the procedure, they should eliminate pain.[68] There is no standard definition of epidural success or failure, and some scholars estimate that the failure rate may be as high as 23 percent or greater.[69]

While Meghan's experience of medical staff dismissing women's concerns may seem extreme, there are also more subtle ways that women felt dismissed or discarded as they birthed their children. Most often women reported knowing intuitively that there was something wrong but being dismissed by medical staff. For example, a week before Joan's third baby was born, she went into the hospital because she felt that "something was off." Despite the medical staff initially dismissing her concerns, she was ultimately proven correct—her amniotic fluid levels were so low as to be dangerous to her fetus.

While the idea of maternal instinct may seem unscientific, recent scientific studies have pointed to evidence that difficulties in childbirth are correlated with a mother having a "gut instinct" that something was wrong. For example, a research team led by midwife and PhD researcher Jane Warland, conducted a survey with mothers who gave birth to stillborn babies as well as those who gave birth to healthy infants. They found that 75 percent of mothers who had stillborn infants experienced an intuitive feeling suggestive of a problem throughout their pregnancy as compared to only 12 percent of mothers who gave birth to healthy infants.[70] While medical practitioners often do listen to patient intuition, it can be difficult to distinguish between pregnancy symptoms—such as being tired and swollen—and those that are more extreme. When medical staff incorrectly reject a mother's concern, hindsight can exacerbate a woman's experience of dismissal and produce trauma.

Here, again, we see how a shortage of time can cause severe injury to women. In their rush to perform Meghan's cesarean, medical staff neglected to review her chart and consider her allergy. They further kinked her epidural and refused to take time to listen and resolve the situation. Rather than taking time to hear Joan's concerns, doctors dismissed her intuition and failed to identify a life-threatening condition. In medical staff's negligence to take time, they are making visible the ways that institutional control over their time limits their ability to successfully perform their jobs. Doctors are rushed. The average doctor sees nearly 2,500 patients annually, 19 people per day.[71] It is this lack of time that causes doctors to fail the women in their care.

The Traumatization of Disrespect

While some women we interviewed experienced trauma that was entirely unrelated to the specific circumstances of their pregnancies or births, the majority of the childbirths discussed in interviews were of an emergency nature, such as spiking blood pressure that required an emergency cesarean or a premature rupture of membranes that led to a helicopter-transfer to a hospital in a larger city. These situations were often *time*-sensitive and required interaction with medical personnel who were not necessarily acquainted with the laboring mother. During such chaotic moments, many women recalled feeling as if they got lost in the shuffle, at best ignored, but at worst, treated or spoken to in ways that felt acutely dehumanizing or infantilizing. Such interactions were frequently referenced as interviewees recounted how their childbirth experiences felt traumatic.

During her pregnancy, Renee had to undergo weekly nonstress tests: tests that monitor a fetus' heart rate and, indirectly, oxygen supply.[72] Because she "carries her weight in her stomach" these tests would take much longer than nurses typically planned. She also found the nurses conducting the test would liberally comment on her weight, telling her she was "too big" and offering "dieting advice." This pattern led her to start to feel self-critical about her weight, fearing it would harm her fetus. She remembers thinking "Fuck you, Renee, for being fat."

The doctors decided to induce Renee and tried several medications, including Cervidil and Pitocin—medicines commonly used to start or expedite labor. She continued to labor when a nurse came in and began to ask insensitive questions about her pregnancy. Renee recalls,

> The very first thing he starts saying is like, "Oh, how did you get pregnant? Did you use a donor? Did you use artificial insemination? Did you, like whatever" and I'm not answering him because it's none of his fucking business. And I'm just like, "Is the baby ok? Like, how's she doing?" and I just keep trying to, like, redirect the conversation. "Because he was really upsetting me. And like he was, asking me about paternity and me and Diane's relationship and if we were married and . . . just all kinds of stuff."

What Renee experienced here is commonly referred to as a microaggression. Microaggressions—interpersonal interactions that cause injury to people of marginalized populations—are a common and continued barrier to healthcare equity for people from historically marginalized groups. The experience of microaggressions leads to psychological stress for its victims and can be exacerbated in the medical setting because of the power differential that exists between providers and patients.[73]

Renee continued to labor, making little progress, and ultimately had to have a cesarean because doctors were concerned for her baby. She was brought to the operating room and, as she received her epidural, medical staff ignored her. She was struck by how insensitive the medical staff was as they ignored her and talked about their lives, "Nothing is being said to me at this point. They're just talking to each other." She remembered them discussing going to Walmart to go shopping. The nurse she was leaning against was "talking about her daughter buying the new trailer." Through it all, Renee remembered, "Nobody was talking to me . . . They give me the shot and then I went numb. Then they started manhandling me and moving me onto the bed and position for the c-section. But nobody is talking to me. Nobody is saying anything."

One last example of how doctor's emotions or actions can be harmful to mothers comes, again, from Ashley. Several years after the experience she shared above, Ashley gave birth to her second child at the same hospital. Her labor was long, about fifty hours. She had switched doctors and was working with a primary care physician who she perceived as "so mad that it was taking so long." The physician exhibited such clear anger that it left her feeling afraid and unsafe, "He got mad 'cause I was not progressing the way he wanted me to . . . He took his gloves off and threw them as hard as he could in the trash can" before storming from the room. This display of anger was unsettling to Ashley, but she was more struck by what happened after her son was born, "After Dennis was born, he said, 'Finally! This is the only baby I've ever wanted to spank.'" Ashley was grateful when the doctor finally left but appalled when, at subsequent appointments or encounters, he proceeded to ask her on dates.

Insensitivity on the part of medical staff exacerbated mother's trauma. This behavior is an indirect consequence of a failure to *take time*. Medical staff behave in ways that are disrespectful, aggressive, hurtful, or infantilizing when they fail to *take time* to consider the impact of their words and actions, when they neglect to mindfully and compassionately interact with patients. In Renee's experience, this manifested in repeated, cruel treatment. For Ashley,

her doctor's lack of *time* resulted in an emotional response to Ashley's lengthy labor and the way that he failed to think about the inappropriateness of his actions toward her during and following her child's birth.

The longer hours expected from rural medical staff and the lack of obstetric resources account for a significant portion of incidences of poor-quality patient-provider interactions. Research on quality of care demonstrates that the size of nursing staff, staff skill variance, and staff training impact quality of care, suggesting that rural health care is of lower quality than that in urban and suburban areas.[74] A shortage of time leads staff to hurry through procedures, often failing to acknowledge the human needs of the patient.

The negative impacts of long work hours are well documented in scholarship on medical practices. Long work hours are associated with increased mistakes, including serious mistakes, higher levels of injuries to patients (such as needle sticks), increase rates of infection in patients, and even increased mortality rates for patients.[75] Current work shifts are also a burden to medical staff themselves. Working long hours causes harm to medical staff's physical health, including cardiovascular disease, physical pain, absentmindedness, anxiety, and irritability, struggling to stay awake while at work, fatigue during their commute and car accidents following their shifts.[76] In effect, working these long hours can leave doctors feeling the effects of exhaustion that mirror drunkenness.[77] This suggests that not only are long work hours stressful for patients and providers alike; they are also deadly.

Efforts have been taken to reduce the number of hours worked by physicians in the United States. For example, in 2003, the Accreditation Council for Graduate Medical Education put limits on work shifts among medical-training programs such that the average number of hours worked per week could not exceed eighty and shifts had to be limited to thirty or fewer hours.[78] In 2011, shifts were reduced to sixteen hours for interns and twenty-eight hours for residents after their first year. Before these measures were enacted, residents often spent over 100 hours per week in the hospital and individual shifts could be 48 hours or more.[79] Yet, as these restrictions were implemented, hospitals did not respond by increasing the volume of hospital staff, which resulted in existing residents having to do the same amount of work in less time.[80]

It may seem clear that hospitals need to reduce the demands placed on medical professionals by reducing hours and hiring additional staff. However, there simply are not enough doctors in the United States to cover the extra work hours. The World Health Organization reports that the United States has an average of 26 doctors for every 10,000 residents. In comparison, countries with better health incomes have a higher ratio of doctors. Germany has 42 doctors per 10,000 residents. Finland has 38. Sweden has 54.[81] This shortage prevents structural change to reduce the work burden currently placed on medical staff.

The shortage of medical staff in the United States is primarily due to costs. Residency programs cost students approximately $152,000 annually. About 26 percent of these costs are covered by Medicare, but doctors graduating from medical school typically have about $180,000 in student loans.[82] Approximately 28,000 doctors receive in-hospital training every year, but the Association of American Medical Colleges estimates the country will see a shortage of 90,000 doctors by 2025 with current staffing practices.[83]

Many solutions have been proposed to solve our shortage of medical professionals. Some, such as the Association of American Medical Colleges, suggest the training of more doctors per year. Others advocate for fixing laws to make the immigration of medical professionals from outside the country easier.[84] In either case, this change requires political will and action to solve this crisis and create the support needed for staff to function.

CONCLUSION

The stories of these women clearly demonstrate how negative experiences with medical staff can exacerbate the trauma they experienced during childbirth. Viewing this from outside the situation, it is easy to empathize with both medical providers and patients. On the one hand, one can clearly see how medical staff would prioritize the health outcomes of the infant and mother over *taking time* to communicate clearly and respectfully. On the other hand, it is easy to understand the mother's perspective. Not knowing the location of one's child, if one's child is going to survive, and or one's own health status would be deeply traumatizing.

According to Foucault, institutional control over human bodies and reproduction is attained via the subtle operations *time*, *structure*, and *routine*.[85] By controlling and limiting doctors' *time* in the name of efficiency and profit, institutions govern and discipline their behavior and the practice of medicine itself. Not only are medical practitioners' bodies and behaviors policed in this way, so too are their patients. In ensuring that doctors never have enough *time*, hospitals and insurance companies may turn a profit, but they do so at the expense of both practitioners' and women's health.

Doctors in the United States, in general, and rural healthcare systems, in particular, are overworked. As a result of the demands of an understaffed healthcare system, doctors are over-extended. This results in patients feeling ignored, unimportant, or, at the worst, overtly mistreated. One might still wonder why the United States is especially plagued by staffing shortages and overworked doctors and why our culture surrounding care seems uniquely harmful to patients. The answer appears to be the perverted financial incentives that operate within the U.S. healthcare system. In short, in our national fear of government overreach and rejection of a universal health care system, we failed to invest in ourselves. The United States spends more than twice per capita what other nations invest in health care, yet has some of the worst health measures in the world. As a result, we do not have the resources to finance the programs and support the people that can and do save lives. Because the United States places its healthcare investment in skyrocketing costs for administrative positions, equipment, drugs, and insurance fees, we lack resources to invest in the staff needed to support patients. People in rural communities disproportionately seek health care in the face of staffing shortages and unequipped hospitals.

When we personally have negative medical experiences, or hear anecdotes from others, we are quick to explain them as the product of a bad doctor or someone having a bad day. Upon further investigation, it is evident that the for-profit structure of the U.S. medical system puts undue pressure on medical providers making it difficult for them to have the needed time to consistently provide high-quality interactions with clients. As compared to their peers in other wealthy nations, doctors in the United States work excruciating long hours, putting themselves and their patients at risk. For women who experience difficult childbirths, the danger posed by long work hours for doctors manifests in negative patient-provider interactions. Medical staff simply do not have the mental capacity to pause, reflect, and connect with their patients.[86] These pressures lead doctors to fail in their communication with patients. All of these behaviors can be traumatizing for mothers.

NOTES

1. "Pregnancy week by week," The Mayo Clinic. Accessed July 7, 2020. https://www.mayoclinic.org/healthy-lifestyle/pregnancy-week-by-week/in-depth/pregnancy/art-20046098.

2. Jeffrey Smith, Richard F. Lowe, Judith Fullerton, Sheena M. Currie, Laura Harris, and Erica Felker-Kantor, "An integrative review of the side effects related to the use of magnesium sulfate for pre-eclampsia and eclampsia management," *BMC Pregnancy and Childbirth* 13, no. 1 (2013): 34.

3. "Magnesium Sulfate Use in Obstetrics," The American College of Obstetricians and Gynecologists. Committee Opinion Number 652. 2016. https://www.acog.org/Clinical-Guidance-and-Publications/Committee-Opinions/Committee-on-Obstetric-Practice/Magnesium-Sulfate-Use-in-Obstetrics.

4. Smith et al., "An integrative review of the side effects."

5. "Treating pre-eclampsia," Health Direct. Accessed June 8, 2020. https://www.pregnancybirthbaby.org.au/treating-pre-eclampsia.

6. Kristin Samuelson, "Post-traumatic stress disorder and declarative memory functioning: A review," *Dialogues in Clinical Neuroscience* 13, no. 3 (2011): 346–351.

7. Mina Abbassi-Ghanavati, James M. Alexander, Donald D. McIntire, Rashmin C. Savani, and Kenneth J. Leveno, "Neonatal effects of magnesium sulfate given to the mother," *American Journal of Perinatology* 29, no. 10 (2012): 795–800.

8. Michel Foucault, *Discipline and Punish: The Birth of the Prison* (New York: Vintage, 2012).

9. Susan Bordo, "Feminism, Foucault, and the politics of the body," in *Bodies and Pleasures,* ed. Ladelle McWhorter (Bloomington, IN: Indiana University Press, 1999), 179–201.

10. Michel Foucault, *The Essential Foucault: Selections from Essential Works of Foucault, 1954-1984* (New York: The New Press, 2003), 306.

11. Michel Foucault, *Discipline and Punish* (New York: Random House, 1977)

12. Foucault. *Discipline and Punish.*

13. Foucault. *Discipline and Punish.*

14. Institute of Medicine. *Employment and Health Benefits: A Connection at Risk.* (Washington, DC: The National Academies Press, 1993); "Our History." Commissioned Corps of the U.S. Public Health Service. Accessed November 17, 2020. https://www.usphs.gov/aboutus/history.aspx.

15. Stephen Redhead and Agata Dabrowska, "Public Health Service Agencies: Overview and Funding (FY2010-FY2016)," U.S. Congressional Research Service. October 13, 2015. https://fas.org/sgp/crs/misc/R43304.pdf.

16. Carleton Chapman and John M. Talmadge, "Historical and political background of federal health care legislation," *Law & Contemporary Problems* 35 (1970): 334.

17. Chapman and Talmadge, "Historical and Political Background of Federal Health Care Legislation," 334–347.

18. Institute of Medicine, "Employment and Health Benefits."

19. Institute of Medicine, "Employment and Health Benefits."

20. Chapman and Talmadge, "Historical and Political Background of Federal Health Care Legislation," 334–347.

21. Institute of Medicine. "Employment and Health Benefits."

22. Institute of Medicine. "Employment and Health Benefits."

23. Institute of Medicine. "Employment and Health Benefits."

24. Institute of Medicine. "Employment and Health Benefits."

25. Institute of Medicine. "Employment and Health Benefits."

26. Institute of Medicine. "Employment and Health Benefits."

27. Chapman and Talmadge, "Historical and Political Background of Federal Health Care Legislation," 334–347.

28. Chapman and Talmadge, "Historical and Political Background of Federal Health Care Legislation," 334–347.

29. Michael Katz, *The Undeserving Poor* (Oxford: Oxford University Press, 2013).

30. Chapman and Talmadge, "Historical and Political Background of Federal Health Care Legislation," 334–347.

31. Institute of Medicine, "Employment and Health Benefits"; Odin Anderson, *The Uneasy Equilibrium: Private and Public Financing of Health Services in the United States, 1875–1965*. New College and University Press, 1968.

32. Paul Starr, "The social transformation of American medicine," PhD dissertation, Harvard University, 1978.

33. "Health Care Crisis: Who's At Risk?" Public Broadcasting System. Accessed November 20, 2020. https://www.pbs.org/healthcarecrisis/.

34. Chapman and Talmadge, "Historical and Political Background of Federal Health Care Legislation," 334–347.

35. Solomon Benatar, "Just healthcare beyond individualism: Challenges for North American bioethics," *Cambridge Q. Healthcare Ethics* 6 (1997): 397.

36. "Health Care Crisis: Who's at Risk?" Public Broadcasting System.

37. Gerard F. Anderson, Peter Hussey, and Varduhi Petrosyan, "It's still the prices, stupid: why the US spends so much on health care, and a tribute to Uwe Reinhardt" *Health Affairs* 38, no. 1 (2019): 87–95.

38. David U. Himmelstein, Robert M. Lawless, Deborah Thorne, Pamela Foohey, and Steffie Woolhandler, "Medical bankruptcy: still common despite the Affordable Care Act," (2019): 431–433.

39. Lorie Konish, "This is the real reason most Americans file for bankruptcy," CNBC. February 11, 2019. Accessed May 24, 2020. https://www.cnbc.com/2019/02/11/this-is-the-real-reason-most-americans-file-for-bankruptcy.html.

40. Stephen S. Lim, Rachel L. Updike, Alexander S. Kaldjian, Ryan M. Barber, Krycia Cowling, Hunter York, Joseph Friedman, "Measuring human capital: A systematic analysis of 195 countries and territories, 1990–2016," *The Lancet* 392, no. 10154 (2018): 1217–1234.

41. Karen Davis, Kristof Stremikis, David Squires, and Cathy Schoen, "Mirror, Mirror on the Wall." *The Commonwealth Fund*. June 2014. Accessed June 6, 2020.

https://www.commonwealthfund.org/sites/default/files/documents/___media_files
_publications_fund_report_2014_jun_1755_davis_mirror_mirror_2014.pdf.

42. "Health Spending," Organization for Economic Co-operation and Development. Accessed June 20, 2020. https://data.oecd.org/healthres/health-spending.htm; Yoni Blumberg, "Here's the real reason health care costs so much more in the U.S.," *NBC*. Accessed Jun 18, 2020. https://www.cnbc.com/2018/03/22/the-real-reason-medical -care-costs-so-much-more-in-the-us.html; Davis, Stremikis, Squires, and Schoen. "Mirror, Mirror on the Wall."

43. Elizabeth Hsu, "Medical Pluralism," in *International Encyclopedia of Public Health*. 2nd Edition, ed. Stella Quah (Academic Press, 2016), 8–12.

44. Elizabeth Rosenthal, *An American Sickness: How Healthcare Became Big Buisness and How You Can Take it Back* (New York: Penguin Press, 2017).

45. Thomas Ricketts, "Health care in rural communities," *Western Journal of Medicine* 173, no. 5 (2000): 294.

46. Michael Ratcliffe, "A Century of Delineating a Changing Landscape," United States Census Bureau, Accessed February 21, 2021 https://www2.census.gov/geo/pdfs/reference/ua/Century_of_Defining_Urban.pdf; National Agricultural Library, "What is Rural?" United States Department of Agriculture. Accessed February 21, 2020. https://www.nal.usda.gov/ric/what-is-rural.

47. Reid Wilson, "Rural poverty skyrockets as jobs move away," *The Hill*. December 5, 2017. Accessed June 18, 2020. https://thehill.com/homenews/state-watch/363415-rural-poverty-skyrockets-as-jobs-move-away; Ryanne Pilgeram, *Pushed Out: Contested Development and Rural Gentrification in the US West* (Seattle, WA: University of Washington Press, 2021).

48. Susan Blumenthal, "The effects of socioeconomic status on health in rural and urban America." *Journal of the American Medical Association* 287, no. 1 (2002): 2; Mark Stephen Eberhardt, Virginia M. Freid, Sam Harper, Deborah D. Ingram, Diane M. Makuc, Elsie Pamuk, and Kate Prager, "Health, United States, 2001, with urban and rural health chartbook," (2001).

49. Jane van Dis. "Editors Note," *Journal of the American Medical Association* 287, no. 1 (2002): 1.

50. Hilda R. Heady, "A delicate balance: The economics of rural health care delivery," *Journal of the American Medical Association* 287, no. 1 (2002): 110–110.

51. Marianne Baernholdt, Bonnie Jennings, and Erica Lewis. "A pilot study of staff nurses' perceptions of factors that influence quality of care in critical access hospitals," *Journal of Nursing Care Quality* 28, no. 4 (2013): 352–359.

52. Roni Jacobson, "Widespread understaffing of nurses increases risk to patients," *Scientific American*. July 14, 2015.

53. Kayt Sukel, "Dealing with the shortage of rural physicians," *Medical Economics,* August 29 (2019).

54. Stuart Heiser, "New findings confirm predictions on physician shortage," *AAMC*, April 23, 2019. Accessed June 7, 2020. https://www.aamc.org/news-insights/press-releases/new-findings-confirm-predictions-physician-shortage.

55. Howard Rabinowitz and Nina Paynter, "Reproductive health care in the rural United States," *Journal of the American Medical Association* 287, no. 1 (2002): 6.

56. Bennett. "Reproductive Health Care in the Rural United States," 5.

57. Trude Bennett, "Reproductive Health Care in the Rural United States," *Journal of the American Medical Association* 287, no. 1 (2002): 5.

58. Bennett. "Reproductive Health Care in the Rural United States," 5; National Women's Law Center. "Below the radar: Religious refusal to treat pregnancy complications put women in danger," Accessed February 5, 2021. https://www.nwlc.org/sites/default/files/pdfs/ibis_factsheet_final.pdf.

59. Patty Robertson. "Career information: Obstetrics and gynecology," *University of California—San Francisco School of Medicine.* April 2013. Accessed July 10, 2020. https://meded.ucsf.edu/md-program/current-students/resources-current-studen ts/advising-and-career-development/career-advisors/career-information-obstetrics -gynecology.

60. Medscape, "Medscape physician compensation report 2019," Accessed July 7, 2020. https://www.medscape.com/slideshow/2019-compensation-ob-gyn-6011337#17.

61. Michael Ollove, "A Shortage in the Nation's Maternal Health Care," The Pew Charitable Trust. August 15, 2016. Accessed July 10, 2020. https://www.pewtrusts .org/en/research-and-analysis/blogs/stateline/2016/08/15/a-shortage-in-the-nations-m aternal-health-care.

62. Kathleen Rice Simpson, "An overview of distribution of births in United States hospitals in 2008 with implications for small volume perinatal units in rural hospitals," *Journal of Obstetric, Gynecologic & Neonatal Nursing* 40, no. 4 (2011): 432–439; Lan Zhao, *Why Are Fewer Hospitals in the Delivery Business?* (Bethesda, MD: NORC at the University of Chicago, 2007).

63. Ollove, "A Shortage in the Nation's Maternal Health Care"; U.S. Census Bureau. "Fast Facts—Idaho." 2019. Accessed October 26, 2020. https://www.census .gov/quickfacts/ID.

64. Marty Makary, *The Price We Pay: What Broke American Health Care—and How.* (New York: Bloomsbury, 2019).

65. Jacqueline Wolf, *Cesarean Section* (Baltimore, MD: Johns Hopkins University Press, 2018).

66. One important type of traumatizing event is not present in this chapter, that of obstetric violence and a failure of staff to obtain consent from mothers. Rather, I have dedicated a full chapter (chapter 4) to this egregious failure of obstetric care and use it to explore how *time, space,* and *routine* operate in concert to impact women in childbirth.

67. Martha Sears and William Sears, *The Attachment Parenting Book* (Boston: Little Brown and Company, 2001).

68. "Pregnancy and birth: Epidurals and painkillers for labor pain relief." Institute for Quality and Efficiency in Health Care. March 22, 2018. Accessed February 21, 2021, https://www.ncbi.nlm.nih.gov/books/NBK279567/.

69. Angukumar Thangmuthu, Ian Russell, and Mak Purva, "Epidural failure rate using a standardised definition," *International Journal of Obstetric Anesthesia* 22, no. 4 (2013): 310–315.

70. Jane Warland, Alexander EP Heazell, Tomasina Stacey, Christin Coomarasamy, Jayne Budd, Edwin A. Mitchell, and Louise M. O'Brien. "'They told me all

mothers have worries', stillborn mother's experiences of having a 'gut instinct' that something is wrong in pregnancy: Findings from an international case–control study," *Midwifery* 62 (2018): 171–176.

71. Lenny Bernstein, "How many patients should your doctor see each day," *The Washington Post.* May 22, 2014. Accessed November 20, 2020. https://www.was hingtonpost.com/news/to-your-health/wp/2014/05/22/how-many-patients-should-your-doctor-see-each-day/.

72. "Nonstress test," The Mayo Clinic. Accessed October 26, 2020. https://www .mayoclinic.org/tests-procedures/nonstress-test/about/pac-20384577.

73. Silva Mazzula and Rebecca R. Campón, "Microaggressions: Toxic rain in health care," in *Microaggression Theory: Influence and Implications*, eds Gina Torino, David Rivera, Christina Capodilupo, Kevin Nadal, and Derald Wing Sue (Hoboken, NJ: Wiley and Sons, 2018), 108.

74. Jennings Baernholdt and Erica Lewis, "A Pilot Study of Staff Nurses' Perceptions," 352–359.

75. Ann Rogers, Wei-Ting Hwang, Linda D. Scott, Linda H. Aiken, and David F. Dinges, "The working hours of hospital staff nurses and patient safety," *Health Affairs* 23, no. 4 (2004): 202–212; Fiona Flinn and Claire Armstrong, "Junior doctors' extended work hours and the effects on their performance: The Irish case," *International Journal for Quality in Health Care* 23, no. 2 (2011): 210–217; Steven W. Lockley, Laura K. Barger, Najib T. Ayas, Jeffrey M. Rothschild, Charles A. Czeisler, and Christopher P. Landrigan, "Effects of health care provider work hours and sleep deprivation on safety and performance," *The Joint Commission Journal on Quality and Patient Safety* 33, no. 11 (2007): 7–18; Pratibha P. Kane, "Stress causing psychosomatic illness among nurses," *Indian Journal of Occupational and Environmental Medicine* 13, no. 1 (2009): 28.

76. Lockley, Barger, Ayas, Rothschild, Czeisler, and Landrigan, "Effects of health care provider work hours and sleep deprivation on safety and performance," 7–18; Kane. "Stress causing psychosomatic illness among nurses," 28–32. doi:10.4103/0019-5278.50721; Marianna Virtanen, Tiina Kurvinen, Kirsi Terho, Tuula Oksanen, Reijo Peltonen, Jussi Vahtera, Marianne Routamaa, Marko Elovainio, and Mika Kivimäki. "Work hours, work stress, and collaboration among ward staff in relation to risk of hospital-associated infection among patients," *Medical Care* (2009): 310–318.

77. Drew Dawson and Kathryn Reid, "Fatigue, alcohol and performance impairment," *Nature* 388, no. 6639 (1997): 235–235.

78. Ryan Park, "Why so many young doctors work such awful hours," *The Atlantic*, February 21, 2017. Accessed July 6, 2020. https://www.theatlantic.com/bu siness/archive/2017/02/doctors-long-hours-schedules/516639/.

79. Park. "Why so many young doctors work such awful hours."

80. Park. "Why so many young doctors work such awful hours."

81. "Density of physicians." World Health Organization. Accessed July 6, 2020. https://www.who.int/gho/health_workforce/physicians_density/en/.

82. Aaron Carroll, "A doctor shortage? Let's take a closer look," *The New York Times.* November 7, 2016. Accessed July 9, 2020. https://www.nytimes.com/2016/1 1/08/upshot/a-doctor-shortage-lets-take-a-closer-look.html.

83. Lenny Bernstein, "U.S. faces 90,000 doctor shortage by 2025, medical school association warns," *The Washington Post.* March 3, 2015. Accessed July 8, 2020. https://www.washingtonpost.com/news/to-your-health/wp/2015/03/03/u-s-faces-90000-doctor-shortage-by-2025-medical-school-association-warns/.

84. Carroll, "A doctor shortage? Let's take a closer look."

85. Michael Foucault, *Discipline and Punish: The Birth of the Prison* (Harmondsworth: Penguin, 1991).

86. Flinn and Armstrong, "Junior doctors' extended work hours," 210–217; Rikinkumar S. Patel, Ramya Bachu, Archana Adikey, Meryem Malik, and Mansi Shah, "Factors related to physician burnout and its consequences: A review," *Behavioral Sciences* 8, no. 11 (2018): 98; Maria Panagioti, Keith Geraghty, Judith Johnson, Anli Zhou, Efharis Panagopoulou, Carolyn Chew-Graham, David Peters, Alexander Hodkinson, Ruth Riley, and Aneez Esmail, "Association between physician burnout and patient safety, professionalism, and patient satisfaction: A systematic review and meta-analysis," *JAMA Internal Medicine* 178, no. 10 (2018): 1317–1331.

Chapter 2

"Worse Than the Birth"

The Trauma Imposed by Space

Kayla experienced traumatic births with both of her children. During our interview, she begins with the story of her eldest, her son. At thirty-eight-weeks pregnant, just as she was about to teach a class, Kayla's water broke. She and her husband went to the birth center where she was to give birth with a midwife.

Unfortunately, in the middle of her son's birth, Kayla's midwife had to leave for a vacation, leaving her with a substitute. After her son was born, he experienced some respiratory problems. The team and her husband all attended to her son, but the substitute was unfamiliar with the birth center and was unable to locate the needed tools. Kayla recalls, "there was just lots of commotion." Meanwhile, Kayla was "losing tons of blood because they were all attending to the baby."

For reasons unknown to Kayla, the substitute midwife decided to leave and abandoned Kayla with the midwife's assistant. The assistant did not feel qualified to deal with the crisis and called in a second assistant and a third midwife. This third midwife arrived, surveilled the situation, and "within minutes" decided "we are going to the hospital."

Kayla, her husband, and their baby rode in their own car to the hospital several blocks away. There they were both admitted, Kayla for blood loss, her son for respiratory problems and low blood sugar. While all of this was incredibly frightening, Kayla recalls that "the really crappy part about all of that was that the third midwife . . . was very, almost aggressive" about not having been at the birth. While Kayla understood that the midwife did not want to be held responsible for the problems that occurred, she felt hurt by the "way she was going about it." In her mind, the midwife had the paperwork, knew the facts of the event, and could have simply shared these with the medical staff without defensiveness.

Kayla also felt that the hospital "treated us like second class citizens because it was an out of hospital birth." She recalls, "They immediately put my son on antibiotics because 'oh, I'm sure he brought some kind of infection from, you know.'" Kayla comments, "It was a birth center. We didn't give birth on the street. Everything was sterile and all the medical equipment was there, and everything was done according to how it was supposed to be done."

In the hospital, Kayla spent significant time alone as the staff attended to her son. Though she did have a few pleasant moments nursing him, she mostly felt exhausted from the birth and blood loss. At one point, she woke up and panicked, "I don't know where my baby is. I have a baby. I need to find my baby." Then she wandered through the halls in a backless hospital gown looking for her son. When she finally found him, she was notified that they were going to transfer him via air ambulance to a Level IV NICU in a city about 90 miles away.

Several hours after her son left on the helicopter, Kayla was discharged from the hospital. It was the middle of the night. She and her husband packed their bags and drove to the city to which her son was taken. As with North Hospital, Kayla found the NICU to be suspicious of them because of their out-of-hospital birth. The staff tested the family for methicillin-resistant Staphylococcus aureus (MRSA), a type of bacteria resistant to antibiotic treatment, and isolated them from the other residents of the ward.

In the end, Kayla's son needed to stay in the NICU for ten days while he was treated for respiratory problems. Kayla and her husband stayed at a hotel several miles from the hospital and spent a great deal of time going back and forth to visit their son during his stay.

Kayla's experience demonstrates how the institutional use of and norms around *space* can cause harm to mothers. Despite the centuries-long tradition of midwifery in the United States, many states prohibit midwives from practicing within hospitals relegating them to out-of-hospital centers and homebirths. In the location of this study, the birth center and hospital are separated by space based on this institutional rejection of the value of midwifery. Kayla was harmed in having to move between these spaces both by the actual physical relocation in space and then further by the disparaging assumptions staff made about the danger posed by out-of-hospital births. Even her third midwife internalized this knowledge and reproduced it in her defensiveness. This operation of power-knowledge served to discipline Kayla and her family, causing unneeded pain.

Chapter 1 briefly discussed how Foucault conceptualizes the operation of power in contemporary society. To summarize, he sees power-knowledge operating through the creation of discourse that defines what is normal, right, and good in a given context. Institutions employ this power-knowledge to control people within their sphere via managing their use of time, space, and routine.

Foucault engages with space extensively in his work. He contends that "In the first instance, discipline proceeds from the distribution of individuals in space."[1] Institutions distribute people in space, placing them in a given location vis-à-vis others. This could be an enclosure—a space shut off from others such as the hospital itself; a partition—a location for an individual alongside others, such as hospital rooms; functional space, such as separating an infectious disease unit from others, or a rank-order—a hierarchy of people, such as doctor-patient. It is through the distribution of space and the location of various bodies within space that people are controlled. Space, like time, is routinized and internalized such that people within these systems come to accept their positions as given or normal.

In this chapter, then, I apply the idea of institutional control through space by looking at two ways that space exacerbates trauma for women. First, I look at the separation of midwifery and hospital care in the United States and the trauma women experienced during transfers of care. Second, I look at the layout of the NICU and how its physical structure harms mothers as it separates them from their infants.

A BRIEF GENEALOGY OF OBSTETRIC CARE

Childbirth in the United States in the 1800s typically took place in one's home, often with a midwife. Women—neighbors, friends, and family—attended births, which were often a time of social connection.[2] Midwives offered few interventions and primarily joined friends in supporting women as they gave birth to their child. While such a setting may sound idyllic, this era of childbirth featured extreme fear of pain and death for the mother or child.[3] The associated fear of childbirth contributed to the medicalization process which succeeded this age of homebirth.[4]

Around the turn of the century, U.S. culture surrounding childbirth came to increasingly medicalize obstetric care in the United States. Childbirth moved from the home to hospitals; under the care of a (woman) midwife to a (man) doctor. By the 1940s, over half of the women gave birth in the hospital. By the 1970s, nearly 90 percent of childbirths in the United States were in hospitals.[5] This transition was first made by wealthier white women who could afford obstetricians and hospital care and were also perceived as weaker and unable to withstand the pain of childbirth. Poor women, immigrant women, and women of color continued to give birth at home with a midwife for much longer.[6]

The medicalization of childbirth was caused by several concurrent factors. Medicine as a profession expanded and hospitals became more prevalent

throughout society. Doctors had earned prestige and used that clout to emphasize the danger posed by childbirth. At the same time, women sought the right
to mitigate the pain associated with childbirth, something that had culturally
been denied to them during this era.[7] Women viewed the right to a painless
childbirth as a way to gain control over the process.[8]

Despite these desires, the transition to doctors was met with cultural
resistance. Many felt that men should not be present during birth and should
not see women's partially unclothed bodies. To accommodate public pressure, doctors limited physical contact with mothers, darkened the room,
used a curtain to prevent them from seeing the mother, and employed
tools—such as a speculum—instead of their hands for exams. In the end,
childbirth became a more private event in exchange for a sense of safety and
pain relief.[9] In turn, midwifery was pushed to the margins, its knowledge
rejected, and deemed inferior and dangerous in comparison to medicalized
obstetrics.

In response to this era of the medicalization of childbirth, women in the
1960s began to consider that giving birth in the hospital was often an alienat-
ing experience. Sterile. Lonely. Far removed from loved ones. Women often
felt disconnected from childbirth itself. From this response, demand for so-
called "natural" birth began.[10]

Adherents of the natural birth movement often critique the medicalization
of childbirth generally and the cascade of interventions that often occurs
specifically. They argue that excessively monitoring infants often leads to
overzealous treatment and unnecessary interventions, such as cesareans.
This movement further argues that women who give birth in hospitals have
reduced control over their births and are often forced to follow the doctor's
agenda rather than their own.[11]

Despite the "natural" birth movement, 98.4 percent of women in the United
States have their babies in hospitals. Just under 1 percent give birth at home
and approximately 0.52 percent do so at stand-alone birth centers.[12] Yet,
out-of-hospital births are increasing nationally, nearly doubling from 35,578
births in 2004 to 62,227 in 2017.[13] In Idaho, where this study takes place,
out-of-hospital births are slightly more common at nearly 4 percent of total
births in 2017.[14] Of women who give birth in hospitals, 27 percent do not use
epidurals or spinal blocks.[15]

In Springfield, midwives are not permitted to practice in hospitals. Women
have the choice of a home birth with a certified midwife, a birth with a midwife at a local out-of-hospital birth center or a hospital birth with an obstetrician. In Greenfield, midwives can practice at hospitals. However, none of the
women in my study had the in-hospital midwife as their primary practitioner,
suggesting that having access to a midwife in the hospital may reduce the
experience of trauma for women.

While the commonality of hospital births could suggest that the natural birth movement has failed to move childbirth out of the hospital, the comparison is actually more complicated. First, there are financial barriers. Insurance typically does not cover out-of-hospital birth and, as a result, cost leads many women to give birth in the hospital. Dr. Marian MacDorman and Dr. Eugene Declercq in their research on birth trends conclude that the fact that increasing numbers of women are selecting to pay out of pocket to give birth out of the hospital indicates the strength of their desire to have demedicalized births.[16] Second, there are legal barriers for home birth practitioners, which make it more difficult for midwives to receive licensing, and they may not be able to practice in all areas.[17]

THE INJURIOUS PARTITIONING OF
HOSPITALS AND MIDWIVES

The spatial divide between the hospital and birth center presents challenges for mothers who need to transfer between them. Alice, for example, was in the middle of giving birth to her baby when her husband "came in and suggested that we think about going to the hospital." She responded by saying, "There's no way. We can't get there." Though the hospital was close, just a few blocks away, she recalls thinking, "I can't get in the car. I can't walk out of this bedroom."

The physical act of transferring also presents logistical challenges for women. Whether women take their own vehicles or an ambulance, they are in the midst of giving birth to their child. They are often naked or near-naked. They are exhausted. Alice recalls, "I was feeling done for . . . I had him grab the car seat and as we were walking out the door, I was in this gown that kinda covered some things. I threw on a bathrobe and it was super warm out that day. So, I'm like buckets of sweat standing by the front door."

Transferring via ambulance involves additional separation and isolation for mothers. Beth was in the middle of giving birth at the birth center when they realized her daughter was breech. The midwife called an ambulance. As soon as they arrived, the center was crowded with EMTs. Beth recalls "too many people came in." They put her on a stretcher and took her to the ambulance. Even that was difficult in the small space. She recalled, "My husband ended up having to bench press one of the couches just to get out of the way." Once at the ambulance, the EMTs told both Beth's doula and husband that they could not ride with her to the hospital. Beth reflected on the process, saying, "It was obviously a short ride but that, honestly, was . . . just a worst experience." She was alone, separated from her husband and doula, in intense pain, and very scared.

The physical separation of midwifery care from hospitals provides injury for the women who are forced to transfer their care during childbirth. This pain is caused by the act of transferring itself and the ways that women are dehumanized in the process of shuffling (in near nakedness and separated from family), but also, such as was the case for Kayla, the hospital staff's internalization of knowledge that devalues midwifery care and out-of-hospital births.

A BRIEF GENEALOGY OF THE NICU

While women in our sample talked at length about the difficulties they faced with obstetric care, for the mothers who spent time in the Neonatal Intensive Care Unit (NICU), this experience was typically the focus of their angst. It is in this case where the disciplinary power of space is evident.

Prior to the 1900s, NICUs were nonexistent. Premature babies or those in need of special care were kept or sent home with their parents and many did not survive. The shift toward hospital care of infants occurred following the invention of an incubator for humans in 1880. Invented by Dr. Étienne Stéphane Tarnier, and first used at the L'Hôpital Paris Maternité, incubators were met with resistance from the medical care industry. People viewed incubators as unscientific.[18] This changed when French doctors recruited Dr. Martin Couney to display premature infants in incubators at the World Exposition in Berlin in 1896. Couney then brought the display to additional exhibitions, most famously the Coney Island Amusement Park. Here he charged visitors $0.25 to see preemies on display. This grotesque exploitation of a vulnerable population served to showcase the success incubation had in regulating babies' temperatures and increasing survival.[19]

Success with incubators led to the recognition that interventions could help infant survival and spurred additional research into medical care for infants. Through the second half of the twentieth century, neonatology emerged as a distinct specialty within pediatrics.[20] The first NICU opened at Yale New Haven Hospital in 1960.[21] Today nearly 500,000 babies in the United States are born premature every year. Medical advances and the services provided in the NICU have increased their survival rate as well as those of babies born with other medical challenges.[22]

In 1976, the March of Dimes published *Toward Improving the Outcome of Pregnancy* which offered suggestions for the creation of the NICU, including facility design. Since that time, other agencies have offered additional recommendations including the American Academy of Pediatrics, the American College of Obstetricians and Gynecologists, and the American Institute of Architects.[23] Most recently, the Committee to Establish Recommended

Standards for Newborn ICU Design published their eighth edition of "Recommended standards for newborn ICU design."[24] These standards deal primarily with the organization of space. They outline the recommended size for rooms (120 sq. ft per baby). They make suggestions about where in a hospital a NICU should be located (on a different floor from, but near the birth ward). They establish standards for the reception area, security procedures, room design, the location of gas, electricity, and hand-washing stations, and much more. These recommendations are not requirements nor are they enforced.

The two NICUs encountered by women in our study are set up differently. The Level IV NICU has three pods, united by a shared reception area. It has a capacity for approximately sixty babies. Every pod has approximately ten rooms, each with space for two infants. Individual rooms have an incubator for babies, a chair and bench for family, and a hand-washing station. They have two concrete walls, one wall of glass with curtains that connects to an adjoining room to permit fast access for medical staff and one wall that is a curtain opening to a central area with a nurses' station. In most circumstances, parents are permitted to stay with their baby except during shift changes twice a day. However, parents cannot sleep or "room in" with their infants. The Level III NICU has room for thirty-eight beds. Babies are roomed in groups of four or five. There is space for each baby to have an incubator and a nearby chair for parents. There is also a hand-washing station. The rooms have three concrete walls and a glass wall that opens to the nurses' station. This NICU discourages parents from continually staying with their infants, preferring, instead, that they come to assist with cares every three hours but not linger. In both hospitals, the NICU is in a secure wing, with a locked door. They are near but on a different floor from the birth center. The hospitals are close to one another and share some medical staff, with doctors and nurses floating between the two NICUs.

THE INJURIOUS SPACE OF THE NICU

The space of the NICU itself can be particularly injurious for mothers. Within the NICU, women face separation from their babies during their child's full hospital stay. Their ability to be in the same space and to spend time with their infant is controlled wholly by hospital staff.

Space causes injury for mothers when their babies are first brought to the NICU. In fact, feeling as though their "baby was taken away" was repeatedly mentioned by mothers as the most traumatizing moment during their care. One person in our study, Lisa, had severe preeclampsia and gave birth to her son prematurely. During her interview, she cried remembering how he was taken away from her immediately following birth, "They took Parker out of me and then they took him to the NICU and then I did not see him for 36 hours."

Once reconnected, seeing one's infant connected to machines, in an incubator, and unable to be held can be particularly difficult for parents. Further harm is caused by the physical distance placed between mothers and their infants during a baby's NICU stay. Unlike other nations, hospitals in the United States do not allow mothers to "room-in" with their babies in the NICU. This practice has several negative implications, one of which is that out-of-town mothers must find places to stay while their babies receive care.

Consider, for example, the experience of Samantha. Samantha spent two weeks with her daughter at the NICU. The hospital had a social worker dedicated to helping families find lodging, but demand was high. The Ronald McDonald House was full, so Samantha stayed in a hotel room across the street from the hospital until she ultimately ended up at the Ronald McDonald House. However, on any given day, she did not know where she would sleep that night. She, in effect, had no space that was hers; simply a litany of spaces that were not. Each day, Samantha had to pack up her room and bring her belongings with her to the NICU for her visits with her daughter; visits that were limited in time and scope, controlled by medical staff. Once she finally had a room at the Ronald McDonald House, Samantha struggled with the new physical distance from her child. Samantha remembers, "The house is like a half a mile away or something . . . There's a shuttle but it stops running at 9:00pm and so I would end up walking and taking a cab because I did not want to miss those cares." Even when she did have a semi-stable place to stay, Samantha could not concentrate on herself or her baby and, instead, had to focus on navigating the complex logistics of visits. She was physically separated from her daughter via space. Consequently, her time with her daughter was further limited by the packing/unpacking and relocating she was forced to endure.

It is worth noting that these structures—the social worker, the hotel, the Ronald McDonald House, the shuttle—are intended to help the women whose babies are in the NICU. However, as is the case in many bureaucratic structures, the systems put in place to solve an issue (where should mothers stay when their babies are in the NICU) become so complicated as to cause further harm.

Residing apart from infants also adds additional logistical and physical challenges for new mothers. Samantha describes her time at the NICU and the exhausting efforts she put into new motherhood, "I would pass out and then get up and set my alarm, get up, pump, put the milk on ice, pass out, or sometimes I would walk it back to the NICU, if I was in the hotel." If, like many European nations, American hospitals allowed mothers to room in with their infants, Samantha would have been able to nurse her baby on command or, at the very least, pump milk and store it without having to navigate significant distance at night.

Beyond causing injury to women upon the initial separation from their infants and the significant distance away from their babies which mothers must stay, women were also harmed when nurses seemingly arbitrarily refused to allow them to hold their infants. For example, many women such as Natalie, recall the anguish they experienced with being inconsistently able to touch their child. Natalie describes the NICU as "worse than the birth," in part, because of rules that are perceived as illogical. She reflected,

> The NICU experience was like that, a lot of times . . . Our experiences with him for a while were just so dependent on the nurse who was assigned to him. Some of them were "yeah, let's do skin-to-skin time, it's the best thing for him" and others were like, "mmm—you need to keep him bundled up because we don't want him to burn calories" . . . I really wanted to try breastfeeding, and some were like, "yeah, it's the best thing for him, let's try it" and others were like, "no, it's going to burn too many calories for him."

Often this unpredictability placed a great deal of pressure on mothers themselves to provide continuity of care for their child. Natalie remembers a nurse telling her to take charge of her child's care,

> There was one nurse who was just super awesome, who we really liked. And she was all about skin-to-skin and trying to breastfeed . . . and when we came in, she would just let us do our thing, and not supervise us. I remember asking, "so some of the nurses don't think we should come in and just interact with him. I'm not trying to like, stir up trouble, but how do you respond?" And she's just like, "oh no, you just come in and start doing it, and if anyone says anything, you just say, "oh no, we breastfeed skin-to-skin, that's what we do." So, we started doing that, and we got a little bit of push-back, but it was a lot better after that, because nobody would be like, "no, you cannot do that!" And we did make a couple of complaints, which I'm glad we did. But it just, it gets exhausting to advocate for yourself, every time you want to see your baby.

This expectation of mothers to demand certain types of care for their child often caused psychological discomfort as they felt torn between doing what they believed to be best for their baby and not wanting to anger the people taking care of them.

NICUs see around eight babies per 100 live births annually.[25] With approximately 8.5 million births in the United States each year, this amounts to 304,000 babies. They are an important source of care for families. Families that need NICU support are disproportionately low-income and from rural communities largely due to high poverty rates, elevated unemployment, and lack of health insurance. People living in rural communities are 9 percent more likely to experience severe disease or death in childbirth.[26]

Memories of the NICU evoke competing emotions for mothers whose children have stayed there. On the one hand, they feel gratitude to the nurses and doctors who saved their child's life. On the other hand, women experience this time as impersonal, inconsistent, and frightening. Mothers recognize that the interventions their child experiences are necessary, they feel unempowered by the way they are treated in the process.

While the physical separation of mothers and infants may be necessary, and it does appear to be nearly exclusively done when there is a medical reason to examine the newborn, it causes severe injury to women. The *space* between them and their infants reflects more than just needed care. For many, it signifies a failure on their part to successfully give birth. For others, the separation is in direct opposition to their instincts as mothers—to provide care for their babies.

CONCLUSION

Like time, space is used by institutions to control people. In the case of traumatic birth experiences, space further injures mothers. The separation of midwifery and medical-based obstetrics creates two worlds of care. It results from and perpetuates societal knowledge that devalues midwifery and out-of-hospital births. Women who need emergency care are then forced to both traverse this space and also bear the brunt of the internalized values of staff. The NICU, too, physically separates mothers from their infants, causing further trauma. The space manifests and reinforces routines that hurt mothers. They are unable to stay with their infants. They are victimized by inconsistently being able to hold their babies.

As I noted in chapter 1, space, time, and routine do not operate separately from one another. Rather, time and space largely control and shape the routines common in a given setting. For example, the routines of caring for infants in the NICU are shaped significantly by the way that medical staff and mothers' time is managed. They are also influenced by the layout of the NICU itself and the separation of mothers from their infants during their stays.

NOTES

1. Michel Foucault. *Discipline and Punish: The Birth of the Prison* (New York: Penguin, 1991).

2. Judith Leavitt, "'Science' enters the birthing room," *The Journal of American History* 70, no. 2 (1983): 281–304.

3. Leavitt, "'Science' enters the birthing room," 281–304; Nancy Dye, "History of childbirth in America," *Signs* 6, no. 1 (1980): 97–108.

4. Leavitt, "'Science' enters the birthing room," 281–304.

5. Katherine Beckett, "Choosing cesarean: Feminism and the politics of childbirth in the United States," *Feminist Theory* 6, no. 3 (2005): 251–275; Jane B. Donegan. "'Safe delivered,' but by whom? Midwives and men-midwives in early America," in *Women and Health in America: Historical Readings*, edited by Judith Walzer Leavitt, 302–317 (Madison, WI: University of Wisconsin Press, 1984); Judith Pence Rooks, *Midwifery and Childbirth in America* (Philadelphia, PA: Temple University Press, 1997); Catherine Scholten, "On the importance of the obstetrick art: Changing customs of childbirth in America, 1760–1825," *Women and Health in America: Historical Readings*, edited by Judith Walzer Leavitt, 426–445 (Madison, WI: University of Wisconsin Press, 1984).

6. Judith Walzer Leavitt, "Birthing and anesthesia: The debate over twilight sleep," *Signs* 6, no. 1 (1984): 147–164.

7. Beckett, "Choosing cesarean," 251–275; Leavitt, "Birthing and Anesthesia"; Donald Canton, *What a Blessing She Had Chloroform: The Medical and Social Response to the Pain of Childbirth from 1800 to the Present* (New Haven, CT: Yale University Press, 1999).

8. Leavitt. "Birthing and Anesthesia."

9. Dye, "History of childbirth in America," 97–108.

10. Beckett, "Choosing Cesarean," 251–275.

11. Beckett, "Choosing Cesarean," 251–275.

12. National Academies of Sciences, Engineering, and Medicine; Health and Medicine Division; Division of Behavioral and Social Sciences and Education; Board on Children, Youth, and Families; Committee on Assessing Health Outcomes by Birth Settings; Backes EP, Scrimshaw SC, editors. Birth Settings in America: Outcomes, Quality, Access, and Choice. (Washington, DC: National Academies Press, 2020).

13. Marian MacDorman and Eugene Declercq, "Trends and state variations in out-of-hospital births in the United States, 2004–2017." *Birth* 46, no. 2 (2019): 279–288.

14. MacDorman and Declercq, "Trends and state variations in out-of-hospital births," 279–288.

15. Alexander J. Butwick, Jason Bentley, Cynthia A. Wong, Jonathan M. Snowden, Eric Sun, and Nan Guo, "United States state-level variation in the use of neuraxial analgesia during labor for pregnant women," *JAMA Network Open* 1, no. 8 (2018): e186567-e186567.–

16. MacDorman and Declercq, "Trends and state variations in out-of-hospital births," 279–288.

17. Debora Boucher, Catherine Bennett, Barbara McFarlin, and Rixa Freeze, "Staying home to give birth: Why women in the United States choose home birth." *Journal of Midwifery & Women's Health* 54, no. 2 (2009): 119–126.

18. "History of Medicine: The Incubator Babies of Coney Island," *Columbia University.* Accessed July 6, 2020. https://columbiasurgery.org/news/2015/08/06/history-medicine-incubator-babies-coney-island.

19. "History of medicine: The incubator babies of Coney Island." *Columbia University.*

20. University of Pennsylvania, Nursing, "Care of premature infants," Accessed November 28, 2020. https://www.nursing.upenn.edu/nhhc/nurses-institutions-caring/care-of-premature-infants/.

21. Louis Gluck, "Conceptualization and initiation of a neonatal intensive care nursery in 1960," In *Neonatal Intensive Care* (Bethesda, MD: National Institutes of Health, 1992).

22. Anne Jorgensen, "Born in the USA: The History of Neonatology in the United States: A century of caring," *NICU Currents,* 2010. Accessed June 20, 2020. https://static.abbottnutrition.com/cms-prod/anhi-2017.org/img/history-of-neonatology_tcm1423-102720.pdf.

23. Robert D. White, Judith A. Smith, and Mardelle M. Shepley, "Recommended standards for newborn ICU design," *Journal of Perinatology* 33, no. 1 (2013): S2–S16.

24. White, Smith, Shepley, "Recommended standards for newborn ICU design."

25. Wade Harrison and David Goodman, "Epidemiologic trends in neonatal intensive care, 2007–2012." *JAMA Pediatrics* 169, no. 9 (2015): 855–862.

26. Katy Backes Kozhimannil, Julia D. Interrante, Carrie Henning-Smith, and Lindsay K. Admon, "Rural–urban differences in severe maternal morbidity and mortality in the US, 2007–15," *Health Affairs* 38, no. 12 (2019): 2077–2085.

Chapter 3

"That's Problematic"

The Trauma Imposed by Routine

We hold our interview in the borrowed second-floor office of a cozy old house that has been converted to a maternal support center in our shared small town. Lisa began the conversation by telling me about her experience while pregnant. She was only twenty-eight-weeks pregnant when she realized that the sickness she felt was not typical of pregnancy. But, because it was her first time pregnant, Lisa worried she was overreacting. At her next appointment, her urinalysis indicated elevated protein levels alongside a high blood pressure reading, signs of preeclampsia. After a second appointment where she exhibited the same symptoms, her doctors still dismissed her concerns, so Lisa transferred her care to another clinic. Her new doctor, astonished at both the protein level and blood pressure, which by then was "really elevated," immediately sent Lisa to the birth center at the local critical access hospital. She spent the next two weeks having nonstress tests every three days.

Meanwhile, Lisa was reading about preeclampsia online and trying self-prescribed food-based remedies to reduce blood pressure in the absence of medication. But these efforts were not enough and, following another nonstress test and urinalysis, she was driven through a snowstorm by ambulance to a large hospital approximately 90 miles away. She was thirty-one-weeks pregnant.

Lisa's time in the hospital, prior to having her son, was a blur of repeated questioning—"do you have visual disturbances? Do you have gastric pain?" Her blood pressure was incredibly high, and she felt very sick as she went to sleep each night fearing that she would not wake up in the morning.

Then, one day, Lisa's vision faltered, and tests indicated that her liver was failing. The nurses called her husband and mother, who were both back at their respective homes, and took her to surgery for an emergency cesarean. Once her son, Parker, was born, medical staff immediately took him to the

51

Neonatal Intensive Care Unit (NICU), and she was unable to see him for the next thirty-six hours. Recalling this part of her birth, Lisa began to cry, "I didn't get the put-your-baby-on-your-chest thing." She shook her head, "I don't remember a lot after that." Meanwhile, Lisa was placed on magnesium sulfate to help reduce her blood pressure. This medication has intense side effects and can make those taking it feel very ill.

When Lisa finally got the opportunity to meet her son, her primary emotion was fear. She recalled, "There's this tiny baby. I was scared of him. He was so tiny." She began to cry again. "You know, this little incubator . . . I couldn't hold him. I couldn't touch him." On that day, she fainted in the NICU and was told by medical staff that she could not return to see her son until she was better.

Once she was strong enough, Lisa began to visit Parker in the NICU as often as possible. In the NICU, infant care times run on three-hour cycles. Lisa attended every care time except for those at 2:30 and 5:30 in the morning because the staff encouraged her to sleep. Meanwhile, the three other babies that shared a room with Parker were suffering from drug withdrawal, having been born to mothers struggling with addiction. Lisa is still haunted by their cries years later.

Lisa recalls that her primary experience in the NICU was a feeling of confusion. The staff rotated frequently and there was little consistency between nurses and doctors attending to Parker. As a result of the constantly alternating staff, the rules Lisa was expected to adhere to were always changing. Some nurses allowed and encouraged Lisa to hold her baby skin-to-skin. Others insisted she leave the baby in the incubator and refrain from touching him. It was torture.

When Lisa would have been thirty-nine-weeks pregnant but was already the mother of a 7-week-old infant, the hospital in her hometown—the very one that transferred her—called to offer her a tour of the maternity ward prior to her birth. Lisa was furious,

> I almost ripped the woman a new one even though I know that it's not her fault. I was like, "Why? What do you mean? You mean for the baby I gave birth to seven weeks ago?" And she was like, "oh I had no idea." I was like, "that's a problem that you have no idea, like you transported me to Greenville, you have no idea? There's nothing in my paperwork that says I already have a baby? That's problematic."

Once home with Parker, Lisa continued to suffer both physically and emotionally. The next seven weeks she bled continuously and, though her doctor assured over the phone that this was normal, she was frightened: "Nobody tells you that you bleed so much after a c-section!" Lisa continued to feel weak and had difficulty with mobility because her legs remained extremely swollen. Yet, she did not receive postpartum medical care beyond the regular two- and six-week checkups. She recalled that the medical team "weren't super worried" but that her platelets were low, her legs were so swollen she "thought [her] skin was going to break open," and she "could barely walk."

On the day that Parker was discharged from the hospital, a social worker visited Lisa and her husband. This was their first meeting and Lisa remembered that "she seemed bothered to talk to us." The social worker administered a postpartum depression survey that is routinely given to all mothers and disappeared. This test is intended to help identify women who may be experiencing postpartum depression, but Lisa lied on the form because she feared "if I don't answer right" the hospital would "take my baby away from me."

Emotionally, Lisa felt isolated from her peers who had had more typical birth experiences and was unable to access the postpartum care she desperately required. Lisa needed to talk with a medical professional about her experience. At the time of our interview, she continued to have nightmares of her son's time in the NICU. The sight of a pregnant woman brings Lisa panic because she fears for that woman and her child's lives.

Lisa's experience was clearly traumatic—she nearly died. Her child was born premature. Yet, there are several instances in which her trauma was exacerbated by failures in the healthcare system. Doctors ignored her symptoms, the hospital called her to tour the birth center weeks after her child was born, her son received inconsistent care, and she was unable to find adequate physical and emotional care postpartum.

In chapter 1, I examined how the U.S. healthcare model was formed, interrogated how one of its key shortcomings, staffing shortages, affects rural health care and provider-patient interactions. I also briefly explored the issue of *time*, and who has control of one's time, to the operation of power more broadly. I explained that in restricting doctors' time in the name of profit, the medical system controls not only doctors' bodies and behaviors but also that of the women in their care. In chapter 2, I applied Foucault's concept of control through *space* and examined the cases of transferring care and the NICU.

Both time and space clearly played a role in Lisa's trauma. She was separated from her infant. Her access to him was restricted both through space and time. But she was also injured by power exerted through *routine*. The hospital called her for a tour as a matter of course, though they had already transferred her to the city. She was unable to access needed care following her son's birth beyond the routine two- and six-week postpartum visits.

In this chapter, I extend this analysis to further explore how institutions use routine to exercise power/knowledge and exert control. I do this by exploring the inhumanity of bureaucracies, the central ways that the bureaucratic nature of certain U.S. healthcare systems fails rural mothers seeking obstetric care. I further explore two ways that women are controlled through the routines built into obstetric care. First, I show how institutions deny women care as a matter of course—routine, habit, or because they always have. Second, I demonstrate that the high infant and maternal mortality rates in the United States also derive from the routines of healthcare.

BUREAUCRATIC INHUMANITY: THE INJURY OF ROUTINE

Perhaps the leading theorist on the topic of bureaucracies is Max Weber. Weber was a German sociologist who viewed bureaucracies as the most efficient and rational style of organizational structure.[1] Weber conceived of bureaucracies as an "iron cage" that dictated the rules to which all people must adhere, limiting individuality, choice, autonomy, and creativity.[2]

Since his writings in the early 1900s, others have further explored the inhuman and inhumane effects of bureaucratic structures. Franz Kafka, for example, in his book *The Trial*, traces the angst, confusion, and pain of a man called Josef K. who is charged, tried, and convicted of a crime without ever having faced a judge, met his accusers, or knowing his alleged crime.[3] Kafka uses this story to interrogate the ways that bureaucracies operate outside of formal rules, instead of following the practice of "negotiated order" or informally developed patterns of behavior (routine).[4]

Political theorist Hannah Arendt also addresses this crisis in her work, *A Report on the Banality of Evil*.[5] Here, Arendt uses the case of Adolf Eichmann's trial for his role as an SS officer in Nazi Germany to examine how ordinary people do horrible things when a structure is established which enables them to do so. Arendt argues that evil happens when people lack the ability to reflectively examine their behavior within a set of structural norms. Philosopher Seyla Benhabib contends that Arendt's concept of the banality of evil may be "better" explained as the "routinization of evil" or its *Alltäglichung* (everydayness).[6]

We can use these theorists' insights to help understand and expand the work of Foucault. As has already been discussed, Foucault argued that power-knowledge produces norms and values to which people acquiesce.[7] People (including medical professionals and mothers) conform to these norms often without awareness or question. Power is exercised over people through control of time, space, and routine (the daily practice or habits built into an institution). Time, space, and routine are not wholly separable, rather they operate with, by, and through one another, deeply intertwined as they discipline actors within an institution. As a matter of course, people continue to perform these acts and follow such norms without question.

In the case at hand, I argue that the bureaucratic structures, or routines, embedded within the healthcare system cause harm to the women operating within them. Doctors, nurses, and other staff, too, are directed by orders, cultural norms, or routines to follow specific paths for care. Such routines can cause practitioners to fail to consider the specific human needs of the individual person in their care.

ACCESS TO CARE

The women in our sample struggled to access the care they needed. They were unable to secure mental health care, postpartum care, and needed treatments prior to and during childbirth. Their access was restricted based on the fundamental practice of rural health care, its rituals and routines as they are enforced by medical staff.

In some cases, this lack of access resulted from a combination of time and routine. Women would have to wait weeks or months to access needed care. Consider, for example, Joan's experience. She reports feeling "okay" the first six months after her child was born. However, then she went to visit a friend in the same hospital where she gave birth to her infant and broke down. She was overwhelmed by negative memories and realized she needed help. She called her obstetrician, and they told her it would be a six-month wait to access care if she was not pregnant. Their practice (routine) was to prioritize obstetric over postpartum care. Given the extent of her trauma and its manifestation in her daily life, Joan knew this was too long to wait. She spent hours on the phone calling other doctors, "I called around and called around. It took a good month to get in to see anybody. That was the part that was like, 'Dude, I need help now. I need help yesterday.' I think that was a struggle I had in this area, was just getting in to see someone." The doctors and medical teams could not make time for Joan, wholly excluding her from receiving care.

The bureaucratic routines of medical care also led to the traumatization of women who were unable to access care needed for them or their babies. One woman in our sample, Samantha, had preeclampsia. She was recovering in the hospital while on magnesium and other blood pressure–reducing medication while her daughter was life-flighted to a NICU 90 miles away. Eventually, she was discharged and able to travel to the city to be with her. She was told by her doctor to regularly have her blood pressure checked and to call him with updates. She recalls,

But no one [in the hospital] would take my blood pressure because I was not a patient. The NICU nurses said they would but they did not have cuffs for adults and so they tried to get cuffs from "mom and baby." They wouldn't let them, and they wouldn't let me go down there and they wouldn't [trails off]. [They said] "you can go to the Emergency Room and check in as a patient." It was fucking ridiculous.

Luckily, a friend, who is a nurse at the hospital, came to visit and was able to take her blood pressure. When she finally called her doctor, her blood pressure had spiked again. Without her friend's intervention, the hospital's unwillingness to take her blood pressure could have been catastrophic.

This added stress for women, such as Samantha and Lisa, could have been avoided, yet the bureaucratic systems, or routines, in which the healthcare system operate, have little room for the human experiences of patients. The for-profit, insurance-based model prioritizes efficiency, speed, and profit and controls women's bodies through time, routine, and space. It offers little in the way of human compassion and accommodation.

Care for mothers typically ends after the baby is born, barring a health emergency and one or two postpartum follow-up doctor visits to make sure the mother is physically healing well. However, many women we talked to desperately required additional postnatal care. This lack of access to care is further explored in chapters 5 and 6.

The inability to access care is especially profound for the women in our sample who were on Medicaid. About half of rural residents use Medicaid, compared to 40 percent of urban residents and even lower rates among suburbanites.[8] The medical care received by people on Medicaid is not equal to those with health insurance. Medicaid recipients are often limited in access to adequate prenatal care and screenings, are more likely to face denied claims, and, when they can access care, are forced to deal with negative stereotypes held by their medical providers.

People with health insurance are more likely than those on Medicaid or who are uninsured to receive preventative care and health screenings.[9] These interventions may prevent negative health outcomes during or after childbirth. For example, prenatal care is associated with reducing the rates of low birthweight babies who, themselves, are more likely to die before their first birthday.[10] Other screenings test for possible genetic abnormalities in infants such as cystic fibrosis or sickle cell anemia. Still others indicate health problems in the mother such as preeclampsia or prenatal diabetes.[11] Prenatal care saves lives. Without adequate coverage, such provisions cost women up to $10,000 per pregnancy (plus an additional $30,000–$50,000 for the birth itself) moreover, premature babies' care cost upward of $500,000 in their first year of life.[12] These are impossible fees for most women in rural America to pay.

One woman in our sample on Medicaid and denied routine aspects of maternal care during childbirth was Candace. A college student when she had her child, Candace remembers being denied an epidural as the most traumatizing moment. She says, "I could not get the epidural because of my healthcare, because I was on Medicaid. Apparently, it was not covered." The clearest memory of her son's birth is the pain she experienced during contractions.

As I mentioned in the introduction, Jessica is not local to Idaho and Washington. Rather, she is from rural Alaska. Like many women in our sample, she too faced a premature birth and a transfer from a critical access hospital to a larger, urban hospital. Due to the fact that so few of the women in our sample were on Medicaid and because Jessica's story transcends any given place, I share her experience here. Jessica has dedicated her life to caring for others. She works with people with severe or profound developmental disabilities in her small town. As with many care-based jobs, Jessica's work pays very little and does not provide employer-based insurance. Instead, she qualifies for and uses Medicaid. When she was twenty-two-weeks pregnant with her second child, Jessica's medical team discovered that her body was attempting to go into pre-term labor. Her cervix was 75 percent effaced. To prepare her infant for premature delivery and stop her labor, she was required to receive a steroid shot and daily injections of progesterone. However, this treatment was not covered by Medicaid. Because of her condition Jessica was unable to continue work, she had to be on bed rest, so her family, already struggling with a low income, was forced to live only on her husband's low salary.

Medicare law is, at best, vague and results in widely desperate coverage depending on the state in which one resides. Coverage includes "pregnancy-related services and services for other conditions that might complicate the pregnancy," "pregnancy-related services are those services that are necessary for the health of the pregnant woman and fetus, or that have become necessary as a result of the woman having been pregnant," and "services for other conditions that might complicate the pregnancy include those for diagnosis, illness, or medical conditions which might threaten the carrying of the fetus to full term or the safe birth of the fetus."[13] While one would likely consider the progesterone shots Jessica required or Candace's epidural to be services covered under this law, inconsistency in coverage and the denial of claims plague those who receive Medicaid support.

One might be skeptical that Medicaid is the problem in these situations and argue that such discrepancies are present throughout insurance-based programs. They would be partially correct. Insurance coverage is similarly unreliable and unequitable. The AARP reports that 200 million healthcare claims (out of a total of 1.4 billion) are rejected annually.[14] Yet, a 2018 study by Gottlieb, Shapiro, and Dunn found that Medicaid had a substantially higher claim denial rate than did Medicare or private insurance.[15]

The disproportionate denial of coverage for women on Medicaid is an example of how routine controls women's bodies. Denied care as a matter of course, their bodies and reproductive power is harmed. This happens suspiciously more often to low-income women and reflects America's social hierarchy which values people with wealth over those in poverty.

Medicaid and its expansion have certainly helped low-income women in the United States access quality health care. The Center on Budget and Policy Priorities estimates that Medicaid expansion saved at least 19,200 lives between 2014 and 2017.[16] Yet people on Medicaid are often treated within the healthcare system as a second tier of patients. People receiving Medicaid fear lower-quality care, often resulting from poor-quality provider-patient interactions due to the stigma associated with Medicaid.

Such stigma is an example of disciplinary power's success. Foucault contends that power is secured in subtle ways, through the management of space, time, and routine, but also through constructing and reinforcing norms and values. In this specific case, cultural values that privilege and prioritize wealthy individuals operate through doctors as they treat women in Medicaid. In our sample, Phoebe explains this practice by remarking on the distinct experiences she had while giving birth to her children, which she attributes to the type of coverage she had. She argues, "I was on Medicaid . . . I was not with my first, I had private insurance . . . I felt like the doctor, the provider, was not very supportive. Like they knew that and so they're different. They treat you different when you have private insurance and when you don't."

Candace further felt that the staff's stereotypes of people on Medicaid led them to be paternalistic toward her. She was listening to Mozart and trying to relax and prepare for an impending cesarean when a night nurse entered her room and told her she needed to put her music away so she could get some sleep. Candace recalls, "She takes my music from me and says, 'You need to sleep.'" Candace found that classical music helped her to relax. She reflects on this infantilizing moment recalling that, "This lady took away my comfort . . . I'm an adult, let me listen to my music!" The nurse's efforts backfired as Candace instead, "stayed up for an hour trying to figure out" how to get to her iPod. "I spent more time thinking about that than resting."

Patients on Medicaid, such as Phoebe and Candace, are correct in their perception of this stigma. Dr. Ellen Wagenfeld-Heintz and colleagues find evidence that doctors do hold biases against patients on Medicaid and often do a poor job treating such clients fairly.[17] As a result, patients often avoid seeking medical care or, in some cases, are told by medical staff not to participate in preventative care programs.[18]

Medicaid is certainly a lifesaving program. But too often the structural forces placed on it via the broader American insurance-based healthcare model cause irreversible, unbearable pain for patients and their families. Unequal treatment of Medicaid recipients is a story of rural America. Rural communities have higher levels of uninsured residents than do urban areas. Rural areas also face high levels of poverty and unemployment. As a result, Medicaid—even with its shortcomings—is an important source of access to health care for rural residents.[19] The failure of Medicaid to provide equal care and coverage to patients is an urgent equity issue. The way that Medicaid operates for those in our sample as they seek obstetric care provides clear examples of how institutions control women's bodies. Through the management of time and control of routine, existing knowledge systems deny women needed access to care.

INFANT AND MATERNAL MORTALITY

The inflexible structure and associated routine care underlying American health care have deadly consequences. The United States has among the highest levels of both infant and maternal mortality rates among wealthy nations.

Dr. Felicia Lester, the medical director of gynecological services at the University of California, San Francisco, contends that maternal mortality rates in the United States are comparably high for several structural reasons. First, the current healthcare system lacks strong continuity of care between women's primary care doctors and their obstetricians or, worse, many women do not have access to primary care to manage the underlying health conditions that make pregnancy and childbirth increasingly dangerous. She claims that women who do not have health insurance are 400 percent more likely than those who do to die from pregnancy-related causes. A second weakness in the current model as identified by Lester is a lack of clear standard procedures for high-risk conditions. As a result, she argues, the quality of care in the United States varies greatly between centers. Finally, Lester points to the lack of clear review systems within American health care. Our structure does not invest in a nationally accessible review system which would enable doctors to quickly examine similar cases and treatments to help with unique cases they face.[20]

These weaknesses as identified by Lester indicate shortcomings in the routine nature of health care. As it is uncritically practiced by routine, women's care lacks thoughtful cross-institutional consideration and review. Women are denied access, and needed procedures do not happen as a matter of course. As a result, women and infants die.

One woman in our study, Kim, lost her baby. At twelve weeks' gestation, doctors diagnosed Kim with a subchorionic hematoma, a blood clot created by excess blood accumulating between the placenta and uterine wall. Subchorionic hematomas are associated with a greater risk of miscarriage, early childbirth, and tearing of the placenta.

At fifteen weeks pregnant, Kim began bleeding heavily. She went to the emergency room, knowing that this was likely a result of the hematoma bursting, something that had happened several times already. However, this time seemed remarkably more severe. Kim recalls, "I'm in a wheelchair, I could hardly stand up" in the waiting room of the emergency room. Before the receptionist would let her through, she insisted on peppering Kim with questions. "I'm losing so much blood and she is like 'and do you smoke?' And, you know, the questions they have to ask, I'm just like 'Give me the fucking ultrasound.' You know? I was so worried."

This time, her baby was okay. As a result of these events, however, she transferred care from the local midwife to her primary care doctor. Still, she struggled. Kim desperately sought information about her condition and her baby's health. However, her doctor was generally unsympathetic and refused to both spend time teaching Kim about her condition and providing extra surveillance for the baby.

Kim again changed doctors, this time to Dr. Miller, a local obstetrician. She found Dr. Miller much more amenable to explaining the situation and recommending care. He told her, "take care of yourself. Don't lift heavy. There are ways you can minimize the risks." Though Dr. Miller also warned Kim that this was a dangerous situation, she valued her time with him because "I just felt that he listened to me."

Four weeks and two emergency room visits for bleeding later, Kim found herself at the hospital again. This time, while the doctors performed the ultrasound, her water broke. "I just knew that's the end." The medical team needed Kim to give birth to the baby. She begged and pleaded for them to "knock me out . . . put me to sleep. I don't want to experience this at all. I don't want to." The staff responded by telling her, "You have to." Kim went through the motions but, "I felt like I was dead, like I was just completely not in that room."

Kim gave birth to her baby in the emergency room. They did not transfer her to the maternity ward. She recalls, "It isn't like we were in the birth suite. We're in an ER, a triage room because it happened really fast." For Kim, this exacerbated the trauma, "I remember that feeling—adding to that disconnected feeling just being in a space that was not even a permanent room. I think there was just a curtain."

After he was born, Kim and her husband were able to hold their son. She remembers feeling hurt by the staff's insistence on calling the event a miscarriage. She says "I've had miscarriages. That was a birth. That was a baby that was born." When Kim recalls the story, she uses the term stillbirth but feels like "it was not quite in the club for that or something."

Kim was ultimately admitted to the hospital. She went through the postpartum care rituals of "the numb thing for your crotch and the ice thing." This caused further pain for her as it made her remember her older sons' births and time in the hospital, making the absence of her youngest all the more poignant.

While the death of her son may not have been preventable, Kim's injury at the hands of the hospital and her doctor's routines was. The Emergency Room receptionist would not permit her access to care. Her primary care doctor refused to discuss her case with her in detail as a matter of routine. The hospital forced her to remain awake for the birth of her son. The staff kept her in a triage room with little privacy during the ordeal. They transferred her to the maternity ward after her son passed. These actions, routine for staff, caused greater injury to Kim.

According to the Center for Disease Control, the United States' infant mortality rate—measured by the number of infants under the age of 1 who die each year—is approximately 5.8 in 1,000.[21] This means that approximately 22,000 infants die annually. National averages, however, mask important class and race differences in the survival rates of children. Among Black Americans, the infant mortality rate is much higher, 11.4 per 1,000. In comparison, the rate among Indigenous Americans is 9.4 per 1,000; for Native Hawaiians and other Pacific Islanders, it is 7.4 per 1,000; for Latinx people, it is approximately 5 per 1,000; for white Americans, it is approximately 4.9 per 1,000; and for Asian Americans, the number is lowest, at 3.6 per 1,000. These disparities result primarily from bias in the healthcare system including unequal access to lifesaving resources and information.[22] Low-income families of all races are more likely than wealthier families to experience the loss of an infant.[23]

Between 2007 and 2016, the maternal mortality rate in the United States increased from 15 to 17 per 100,000 births, to approximately 700 per 100,000.[24] Recent news stories have featured the experience of tennis star Serena Williams, who nearly died following the birth of her daughter, Olympia, and drawn new attention to this issue. Approximately twenty-four hours after giving birth to Olympia via cesarean, Williams experienced a pulmonary embolism—a blood clot in her lungs—a complication that occurs in approximately 1 out of 1,000 women postpartum.[25] Williams had a known history of clotting that was not considered during her daughter's birth, despite her insistence, illustrating Lester's contention that the United States lacks communication across institutions. Following her embolism, Williams then faced a series of other emergencies: her cesarean scar opened from her coughing, doctors found a massive blood clot (hematoma) in her abdomen and, as a result, she had to undergo another surgery.[26]

William's experience also drew attention to the disproportionate number of women of color who die during childbirth or shortly afterward. Black and Native women are two to three times more likely to die from causes related to childbirth than are white women.[27] Low-income women, those with chronic conditions, and those who lack access to adequate health care are also more likely to die due to pregnancy-related causes.[28]

It is no accident or coincidence that maternal and infant mortality rates are higher among populations of color. This, too, is an example of how the state controls bodies and reproductive power. As a nation rooted in white supremacy, the United States has long viewed bodies of color as discardable.[29] This is simply another example of how institutions function in subtle ways to carry out these broader systems of power.

CONCLUSION

The routinization of health care results in women being unable to access needed care outside the routine practices of obstetrics, such as postpartum care or unique care in the case of miscarriage and stillbirth. Furthermore, the U.S. model of insurance-based health care perpetuates existing inequalities between lower-income and wealthier residents whereby Medicaid recipients receive less care, lower-quality care, and face unfair and insurmountable stigma from providers. Finally, the routines of health care, and their reflection of unequal ideological foundation, results in both high and disproportionate cases of maternal and infant death.

These failures are not accidental. Rather, they reflect the broader systems of knowledge and power in the United States which are reproduced and enforced within its institutions. Women lack access to care, experience the trauma of separation from their infants, and face death because they are not valued. This is particularly true of low-income women and women of color reflecting centuries-old systems of white supremacy, capitalism, and misogyny.

In the next chapter, I use the example of obstetric violence to demonstrate how all three forms of institutional and ideological control (time, space, and routine) operate in concern to hurt mothers. In doing so, I trace the ideological foundations which give rise to structural abuses of power and violence against mothers and demonstrate their operation in the present using the stories of the women we interviewed.

NOTES

1. Max Weber, *Economy and Society: An Outline of Interpretive Sociology* (University of California Press, 1978).

2. George Ritzer, *Enchanting a Disenchanted World: Revolutionizing the Means of Consumption*, 2nd ed. (Pine Forge P, 2004); Ashworth, Rachel, George Boyne, and Rick Delbridge, "Escape from the iron cage? Organizational change and isomorphic pressures in the public sector," *Journal of Public Administration Research and Theory* (2007).

3. Franz Kafka, *The Trial* (New York: Tribeca Books, 2011).

4. Hodson, Randy, Andrew W. Martin, Steven H. Lopez, and Vincent J. Roscigno, "Rules don't apply: Kafka's insights on bureaucracy," *Organization* 20, no. 2 (2013): 256–278.

5. Hannah Arendt, *Eichmann in Jerusalem: A Report on the Banality of Evil* (New York: Penguin, 2006).

6. Seyla Benhabib, "Hannah Arendt and the redemptive power of narrative," *Social Research* (1990): 167–196.

7. Michel Foucault, *Discipline and Punish* (New York: Penguin, 1991).

8. Katy Backes Kozhimannil, Julia D. Interrante, Carrie Henning-Smith, and Lindsay K. Admon, "Rural-urban differences in severe maternal morbidity and mortality in the US, 2007–15," *Health Affairs* 38, no. 12 (2019): 2077–2085.

9. Institute of Medicine (US) Committee on the Consequences of Uninsurance. Care Without Coverage: Too Little, Too Late. Washington (DC): National Academies Press (US); 2002. 3, Effects of Health Insurance on Health. Available from: https://www.ncbi.nlm.nih.gov/books/NBK220636/.

10. Cheryl A. Fuller and Robin Gallagher, "What's happening: Perceived benefits and barriers of prenatal care in low income women." *Journal of the American Association of Nurse Practitioners* 11, no. 12 (1999): 527.

11. "Prenatal Tests," March of Dimes. Accessed June 5, 2020. https://www.marchofdimes.org/pregnancy/prenatal-tests.aspx.

12. Leana Wen, "I'm Pregnant. What would happen if I could not afford health care?" NPR. March 11, 2017. Accessed May 24, 2020. https://www.npr.org/sections/health-shots/2017/03/11/519416036/im-pregnant-what-would-happen-if-i-couldnt-afford-health-care.

13. 42 CFR § 440.210. Required services for the categorically needy. https://www.law.cornell.edu/cfr/text/42/440.210.

14. Caroline Mayer, "The Health Claim Game," *AARP Magazine.* Nov/Dec 2009. https://www.aarp.org/health/medicare-insurance/info-09-2009/health_claim_game.html.

15. Joshua D. Gottlieb, Adam Hale Shapiro, and Abe Dunn, "The complexity of billing and paying for physician care," *Health Affairs* 37, no. 4 (2018): 619–626.

16. Aviva Aron-Dine, "New research: Medicaid expansion saves lives," Center on Budget and Policy Priorities. November 6, 2019. Accessed May 24, 2020. https://www.cbpp.org/blog/new-research-medicaid-expansion-saves-lives.

17. Dr. Ellen Wagenfeld-Heintz, Victoria C. Ross and Keon-Hyung Lee, "Physicians' perceptions of patients in a county sponsored health plan," *Social Work in Public Health*, 23, no. 1 (2007): 45–59, DOI: 10.1300/J523v23n01_03.

18. Heidi Allen, Bill J. Wright, Kristin Harding, and Lauren Broffman, "The role of stigma in access to health care for the poor," *The Milbank Quarterly* 92, no. 2 (2014): 289–318.

19. Jack Hoadley, Joan Alker, and Mark Holmes, "Health insurance coverage in small towns and rural America," Georgetown University Center for Children and Families and the University of North Carolina. NC Rural Health Research Program. Accessed September 9, 2020. https://ccf.georgetown.edu/wp-content/uploads/2018/09/FINALHealthInsuranceCoverage_Rural_2018.pdf.

20. Felicia Lester, "Why is Maternal Mortality so High in the U.S.?" University of California—Berkeley. Accessed June 6, 2020. https://www.berkeleywellness.com/healthy-community/health-care-policy/article/why-maternal-mortality-so-high-us.

21. Center for Disease Control, "Infant Mortality," March 27, 2019. https://www.cdc.gov/reproductivehealth/maternalinfanthealth/infantmortality.htm.

22. Khiara Bridges, *Reproducing Race* (Berkeley: University of California Press, 2011).

23. Xiaojia He, Luma Akil, Winfred G. Aker, Huey-Min Hwang, and Hafiz A. Ahmad, "Trends in infant mortality in United States: A brief study of the southeastern states from 2005–2009," *International Journal of Environmental Research and Public Health* 12, no. 5 (2015): 4908–4920; Laura Briggs, *Reproducing Empire: Race, Sex, Science, and US Imperialism in Puerto Rico*, vol. 11 (Berkeley, CA: Univ of California Press, 2002).

24. "Racial and ethnic disparities continue in pregnancy-related deaths," Center for Disease Control. Accessed October 10, 2020. https://www.cdc.gov/media/releases/2019/p0905-racial-ethnic-disparities-pregnancy-deaths.html.

25. Louise Simcox, Laura Ormesher, Clare Tower, and Ian A. Greer, "Pulmonary thrombo-embolism in pregnancy: diagnosis and management." *Breathe* 11, no. 4 (2015): 282–289.

26. Serena Williams, "Serena Williams: What my life-threatening experience taught me about giving birth," *Cable News Network.* February 20, 2018. https://www.cnn.com/2018/02/20/opinions/protect-mother-pregnancy-williams-opinion/index.html.

27. Center for Disease Control, "Racial and Ethnic Disparities."

28. Michael Ollove, "A showing number of U.S. women still die of childbirth. California is doing something about that," *Washington Post.* November 4, 2018. https://www.washingtonpost.com/national/health-science/a-shocking-number-of-us-women-still-die-from-childbirth-california-is-doing-something-about-that/2018/11/02/11042036-d7af-11e8-a10f-b51546b10756_story.html.

29. Dorothy Roberts, *Killing the Black Body* (New York: Vintage Books, 1997).

Chapter 4

"Open Your Legs"

Time, Space, Routine, and Obstetric Violence

Though not employed as a nurse, Erica attended nursing school. While there, she witnessed several unprofessional events including nursing students making comments about "ugly" babies, doctors asking women to "open [their] legs" because "that's how you got this way," and other cruel treatment of mothers. This experience led Erica to decide to have an out-of-hospital birth at a local birth center.

The birth of Erica's daughter began with a police escort from the rural town in which she lived to the out of hospital birth center in a slightly larger town about 15 miles away. She delivered her daughter in the summer, the season of road work, and was stuck en route to the birth center because of the construction. She and her husband called the police for help and, after being evaluated by a team of EMTs, Erica turned down an expensive ambulance ride she could not afford and was instead led through construction by police.

After safely arriving at the birth center, Erica spent the next several hours in labor. Erica recalls feeling grateful for the warmth and support she experienced from her midwife, doula, and husband while there. In particular, she felt grateful that her midwife respected her body, "She never did it without asking. Everything was always with my permission and it was amazing" and that everyone trusted Erica's intuition about her body.

This intuition proved important when, after laboring for some time, Erica felt that something was wrong. She told her midwife who checked the baby's heart rate and then conducted a consensual cervical check. The midwife continued to perceive that things were proceeding as they should, and Erica began to push. Erica was able to feel her daughter move up and down the birth canal. Suddenly, the midwife demanded that Erica stop pushing. She realized that the baby was breech—she was positioned to be born butt or legs first—and Erica would be unable to deliver her at the birth center. By this point, Erica's body felt it "had to push" and Erica fought to resist while her midwife called an ambulance.

Thirty minutes later, the ambulance finally arrived. She recalls feeling severely mistreated by the EMT team, "those bastards made me walk out to the ambulance . . . I was naked from the waist down." Ultimately, they gave her a robe, put her on oxygen, and transported her to the hospital a few short blocks away.

Once she arrived at the hospital, Erica felt enveloped in chaos. Immediately the staff placed an IV without asking; the first she had had in her life. The room quickly filled. In her words, "there was like a billion people in my room," which was the opposite of her desire for a small, intimate birth. Instead, numerous people swirled around her while others watched from across the room. In fact, the ambulance team never left. They stood in the doorway to Erica's hospital room and observed. For Erica, it was very difficult to have people placing IVs and monitoring her without talking to her about their actions. Her anger about the process is evident as she recalls, "nobody really told me what they were doing. They just did shit to me." The medical team placed her feet in stirrups, which she resisted, saying "I got to get up onto my hands and knees." When she tried to move, the medical team "literally pushed me back down and told me I could not. They pushed me back down on the bed. I was so pissed but I could not do anything. There was eight billion of them and one of me."

The trauma of losing agency was exacerbated for Erica, because her husband and midwife had also been displaced in the chaos. She recalls her husband "being thrown into the corner of the room" where they could not talk or even "communicate through looks because there's people just buzzing around me." Luckily, her doula intervened, and her husband was ultimately able to support her through the rest of her delivery.

Erica was then given nitrous oxide, an analgesia, by the doctor, which she did not want, fearing side effects. She remembers the panic around her need to push because the medical team had lost the baby's vital signs and feared she was in distress. Finally, Erica succeeded in delivering her child and felt her body tear as she pushed, recalling "it was the worst part of my entire labor." After her daughter was born, the doctor immediately clamped the umbilical cord, despite Erica's request for delayed clamping. The medical team then "whisked Arianna away" without telling Erica how her daughter was doing nor letting the two meet.

The doctor then gave Erica the drug Pitocin to help her body expel the placenta—again, without her consent. The administration of the drug felt like a huge violation, "I remember looking up and seeing them hook it up and I was like 'son of a bitch, they're giving me Pit' . . . I had nightmares through my pregnancy . . . I was afraid to go to the hospital and they gave me fucking

Pit. I really wanted my body to do it. It was really important for me that my body do everything it needed to do."

Meanwhile, two other horrors were unfolding for Erica. First, the audience that attended her birth continued to stand in the room, where she was naked from the waist down. More importantly, her daughter was being resuscitated and the medical team asked her to call out to Arianna. She recalls, "I remember laying there. I could not see what was going on and there's lights in my face and there's people buzzing around. I remember saying 'Arianna, Arianna, I'm over here. Mommy's over here. Arianna, you're okay Arianna.'" Except for Erica and her husband's calls to Arianna, the crowded room was silent, "It was really quiet. It was kind of scary. I did not know what was happening because no one told me."

Erica's placenta was finally delivered, and Arianna perked up. The obstetrician began to stitch her torn perineum—the space between the vulva and anus. As he finished, Erica recalled, "All of the sudden, without warning, he reaches up inside of my uterus and does something and I almost kicked him in the face." The doctor reported that he was removing blood clots, to which she replied, "warn me, I'm not numb." She feels this was an excruciating violation and recalls, "There was no warning. He just reached his big man-hand up inside of my uterus. I understand a baby just came out of there and there's some room in there right now, but it's still my fucking uterus. You're inside an internal organ. You don't just go in and massage somebody's liver. Why would you do that to my uterus without telling me? . . . I was so mad at him for that."

Finally, people cleared out of the room. Erica was able to focus on her new baby, who immediately turned to nurse. Things seemed to be going well until medical staff determined her baby was jaundiced, and Erica was diagnosed as having cystocele and rectocele—conditions in which the tissue between the vagina and bladder or vagina and rectum is damaged.[1] This condition continues to affect her ability to pass urine and have sex years later.

While Erica feels eternally grateful to her obstetrician for allowing her to deliver a breech baby vaginally, she remains scarred by him "reaching up inside" of her and administering Pitocin without her assent. Reflecting on her experience, she recalls "the doctor should have asked my permission before sticking his hand in my uterus." Now, pregnant again, Erica is terrified that she will, again, have her requests ignored and experience things without her agreement. Erica's experience was objectively fraught with difficulty—she experienced a surprise breech birth, a transfer to the hospital, and repeatedly had her requests denied. However, when she looks back at the experience, it is the fact that her doctors failed to obtain consent that most haunts her.

Globally, and especially thanks to the activism of women throughout South America, experiences such as Erica's are becoming known as obstetric violence, a form of gender-based violence. Obstetric violence can include forced surgeries (including cesareans, episiotomies, or coerced sterilizations), any other forms of nonconsensual procedures, sexual assault (including vaginal penetration such as Erica experienced, physical examinations, or the so-called "husband stitch"—an extra stitch sewn during the repair process following a vaginal birth that is purported to tighten the vagina and improve male pleasure during vaginal intercourse), bodily restraint, bullying, or abuse.[2] Erica's and others' birth experiences illuminate how, far from being an experience distinct for women in the global south, obstetric violence is very much institutionalized in the U.S. healthcare system. In this chapter, I look at the issue of obstetric violence in the United States and the structural and cultural forces that allow it to continue. I pay particular attention to the topic of consent, the history of informed consent in medical care, and the reasons for which doctors continue to violate a woman's right to informed consent during medical care.

CONTROL OF WOMEN'S BODIES

In a series of lectures during the 1970s, French philosopher Michel Foucault repeatedly addressed the ways that the state exerts sexual control to achieve state power.[3] Through what Foucault calls biopower, the state establishes both explicit practices but also coercive and invisible norms and values that reinforce racialized and gendered hierarchies via reproduction. Said more simply—the state establishes a value system under which the material conditions of birth are created and certain bodies are permitted to reproduce while others are not. This process is rendered nearly invisible as it is manifest through deeply conditioned knowledge systems which people accept without question. These ideologies are then unthinkingly reproduced by actors within its system in ways similar to that of the bureaucracies.

Erica's case presents a clear example of how a doctor may internalize the knowledge of a society and reenact it through what they view as normal or routine. Perhaps due to a shortage of time or her spatial move from the birth center, the doctor presiding over Erica's case failed to question the appropriateness of an audience attending her birth. He thought nothing of administering medicine nor touching her body without consent. The habitual practices, or routines, of the situation drove his behavior. He is unlikely to even know that Erica is upset or wounded by his behavior during her birth.

Women's bodies have long been sites of state control and ethnic violence. Anthropology professor Ann Laura Stoler, for example, explains how women's bodies were controlled in ways that both created and maintained racial hierarchies and national boundaries.[4] Control over women's reproduction has served as one of the most consistent and barbaric methods of genocide and eugenics programs in both the United States and the world more broadly.

It is this context in which the continued practice of obstetric violence needs to be understood. These values which dictate whose bodies are worth reproduction, which bodies are worthy of respect, and who is a human worthy of dignity operate in the cultural shadows. They emerge in glimpses through the examination of abuses against women's bodies. As we trace this history in the United States, we see clear patterns reflecting the social hierarchies operating in the United States. Women generally, but especially women of color and working-class women, are disproportionately the victims of historic and continued reproductive violence. At first, this system of social values was explicit through such practices as the eugenics movement, described below. In the present, they continue but their cultural roots are distorted and rendered invisible to those who serve as actors in their reproduction.

Genealogy of Informed Consent and Obstetric Abuse

The current power-knowledge systems, which permit the continuation of obstetric violence, become visible through an examination of the history of the U.S. eugenics movement. A movement which, over the course of half a century, forcibly sterilized over 70,000 women. As with all systems of biopower, including state reproductive violence, not all women were (are) equally targeted. Rather, it was (is) women of color, poor women, and those with disabilities who met (meet) the fate of this barbaric practice. While not the only form of obstetric violence, non-consensual or forced sterilizations are certainly among the most egregious. As such, they provide an important entrance to the history of informed consent in the United States.

In the first half of the twentieth century, the United States welcomed what had become known as the eugenics movement. The movement centered itself on contemporary ideas of Mendelian genetics, which suggested that certain characteristics such as criminality, a lack of moral ethics, and other "undesirable" traits were rooted in one's genetic composition. The term itself was coined by Sir Francis Galton and sought to encourage births among "desirable" peoples and discourage propagation among "undesirable" populations.[5] In the United States, these convictions took hold quickly and firmly because they resonated with cultural values of the time. This was the so-called "Progressive Era" in U.S. history in which the values of the Victorian era (modesty, celibacy) merged with newly embraced scientific "advances."[6] At the time (and in the present), white men controlled the power structures in U.S. institutions (legal, political, medical, etc.). This effectively led to their perceptions of a person's worthiness being encoded into the practice of medicine and obstetrics, whether intentional or not. One example is the creation of compulsory sterilization laws.[7]

In 1907, Indiana created the first law regarding compulsory sterilization in the United States.[8] These policies quickly spread to other states and by 1926 twenty-three states had laws regarding sterilization. Eighteen of those required sterilization for people deemed "mentally defective" or who had committed certain types of crimes. Three other states had laws that outlined procedures for both voluntary and involuntary sterilization. Among those with voluntary sterilization laws, only one (Idaho) required consent from a patient, making them effectively involuntary.[9]

The people targeted for forced sterilization were those deemed by white men in power to be "undesirable." This included, but was not limited to, people with developmental disabilities/diverse abilities, those with mental health challenges, people who had committed certain crimes, those who were poor, gay people, immigrants, and populations of color.[10] Between the 1920s and 1970s, nearly 70,000 people were sterilized in the United States under these policies.

In 1927, compulsory sterilization laws were upheld in the infamous U.S. Supreme Court decision in *Buck v. Bell*. In an eight-to-one decision, the court ruled that existing laws regarding forced sterilization of people with development disabilities were constitutional. In his argument, Justice Oliver Wendell Holmes wrote, "It is better for all the world, if instead of waiting to execute degenerate offspring for crime, or to let them star for their imbecility, society can prevent those who are manifestly unfit from continuing their kind."[11]

As the practice unfolded so too did the ways that women were targeted with compulsory sterilization. In some cases, women were obligated by courts.[12] In others, women were tricked. Andrea Smith, professor of Ethnic Studies at the University of California—Riverside, in her book *Conquest: Sexual Violence and American Indian Genocide*—tells the stories of countless Native women given hysterectomies without their consent. She shares cases of women who were told they would serve as a form of temporary birth control, others who sought care for headaches or tonsillitis and were sterilized as false treatment.

Despite most states repealing their laws in the 1970s, the practice and celebration of coerced sterilization as a measure of controlling "undesirable" populations continued. In 1979, 70 percent of the hospitals that performed sterilizations of women on Medicare failed to secure adequate informed consent in the process.[13] Indian Health Services, the main provider of medical care for Native people, is responsible for most of this violence against indigenous women. In 1976, the General Accountability Office (GAO) estimated that approximately 5 percent of Native women in parts of New Mexico, Arizona, Texas, and Oklahoma had been sterilized without their consent. Some estimates put the numbers in Oklahoma at closer to 25 percent. In fact, in Oklahoma during this time, all the "pureblood women of the Kaw tribe" were sterilized.[14]

Unfortunately, this is just one example of the way that women of color have been the primary victims of the ongoing medical mistreatment of women. Other examples include the testing of birth control on women in Puerto Rico without clear consent as well as forced sterilizations of approximately one-third of Puerto Rican women in the 1960s, of Mexican women in Los Angeles in the 1970s and of Black women throughout the south and especially in North Carolina.[15]

From this history, it is clear that informed consent has not long been an ethical requirement for medical practitioners. It was not until 1957 with the court decision in *Salgo v. Leland Standford, Jr. University Board of Trustees* that a requirement for doctors to provide adequately informed consent was advocated for by law.[16] The understanding of informed consent evolved over the next fifteen years or so ultimately culminating in the 1972 case *Canterbury v. Spence* in which the Judge argued that "[t]he patient's right to self-decision shapes the boundaries of the duty to reveal. That right can be effectively exercised only if the patient possesses enough information to enable an intelligent choice."[17]

Changes in U.S. values informed this shift in medical practice. As civil rights, individual liberties, and equity rose to the forefront throughout the 1960s and 1970s Civil Rights Movement, the moral duty surrounding medical practice was impacted in ways similar to other institutions.[18] Despite this cultural shift, by and large doctors feared these new policies and felt them antithetical to their ability to perform their jobs.[19]

On the coattails of this change in the ethical boundaries of consent, in 1977, the International Childbirth Education Association, under the guidance of Doris B. Haire, issued "The Pregnant Patient's Bill of Rights." This document includes sixteen rights of childbearing women, primarily those rights associated with informed consent.[20] As laws regarding informed consent passed throughout the 1950s, 1960s, and 1970s, women, in general, and women of color, in particular, were largely excluded from their reach. Even today, women in childbirth continue to face nonconsensual interventions and obstetric violence.

Laws on the issue of informed consent in medical care differ by state, are vague, and often exclude the need for informed consent in two situations: when "immediate treatment is needed to preserve the [mother and child's] life" and when mothers have signed a consent waiver.[21] For example, in Idaho, where most of the women in our sample live, the law follows what is called the "professional" standard whereby informed consent is defined and classified by what doctors traditionally offer. Other states, including Washington, where the remaining women we talked with reside, follows the "patient" standard whereby consent is determined based on what a "reasonable patient" would "expect to be told prior to making a decision about treatment."[22] Informed consent not only involves assent from patients but also requires that patients are able to understand relevant information, the implications of treatments and their alternatives, and the ability to make a voluntary choice.[23] In the next two sections, I will explore the contemporary prevalence of obstetric violence in the United States and the cultural and structural reasons for its persistence.

NONCONSENT IN THE PRESENT

Erica's experience, outlined at the beginning of this chapter, is riddled with incidences of obstetric violence.[24] She is given medication without being told it would be administered. An audience watched her birth, without her consent. She was physically restrained, despite her protests to the contrary. Her doctor failed to notify Erica that he would be penetrating her while manually removing blood clots. The list of offenses is long and deeply traumatizing to Erica. Unfortunately, her experiences remain all too common in obstetric medicine.

The frequency with which obstetric violence occurs is difficult to measure. Women rarely report these events, perhaps as a result of embarrassment or fear of being stigmatized, or maybe because they perceive such unjust treatment as part and parcel of having a baby. Indeed, women often accept or dismiss their mistreatment due to the common perception that childbirth is successful if it produces a healthy baby.[25] Regardless of the reasons, women often feel like their experience is unworthy of report or complaint.[26] This is, perhaps, best viewed as an internalization of the ideological systems of misogyny underlying violence against women's bodies, which constitute Foucault's meaning of biopower. As actors within the social hierarchy, the institutional practices of birth in the U.S. health system instills in women that their voices and, in truth, their bodies do not matter.

The ongoing devaluation of women is highlighted in the fact that the state of California continued to use state monies to sterilize women in prisons until at least 2010.[27] The Center for Investigated Reporting estimates that nearly 150 women were sterilized in California prisons between 2006 and 2010 just after they gave birth. Beyond California prisons, approximately 1,400 people were forcibly sterilized in California while giving birth between 1997 and 2013.[28] One woman, Kelli Dillon, is the focus of Erika Cohn's documentary *Belly of the Beast.* Dillon was imprisoned at the age of 19 when her partner died as she defended herself against his abuse. At age 24, Dillon was told by doctors that she needed to have surgery for a cyst. Instead, they gave her a hysterectomy. The doctors never told her, she only found out about the sterilization from her lawyer.[29] California outlawed the practice of forcing women to have sterilizations as a form of birth control in prisons in 2014.[30]

The victims of forced sterilization continue to be predominantly women of color. In October of 2020, a whistleblower alleged that at least five women in Immigration and Custom Enforcement (ICE) custody underwent coercive sterilizations over a two-month period in 2019.[31] The total number of women affected is currently unknown pending a Senate investigation.[32] Regardless of the final number, forced sterilization continues in the United States, against all ethical, legal, and cultural standards.

Beyond the atrocious yet narrow scope of sterilization, we have some insight into the frequency of which obstetric violence occurs thanks to the 2014 "Maternity Support Survey Report." This project asks nurses, doulas, and childbirth educators in the United States and Canada to evaluate the care and beliefs of others in their place of work. According to this survey, only 48.7 percent of nurses, doulas, and childbirth educators believe that practitioners where they work obtain informed consent for each procedure. Seventy-one percent had witnessed a practitioner tell a woman her baby would die if she did not consent to a procedure, a possible form of coercion. Over 86 percent said they had witnessed practitioners conduct procedures without mothers having a choice or time to consider what was being done, raising questions about whether or not informed consent was obtained. Over half (52.2%) had seen practitioners violate the explicit wishes of women in their care.[33] Said simply, obstetric violence—understood as non-consensual, even coercive, forms of intrusive medical practices—is common and widespread. It is routine.

One of the best documented form of obstetric violence treatment of women is the administration of nonconsensual pelvic exams. For example, on February 17, 2020, Emma Goldberg, a reporter for the *New York Times* published a story called "She Did Not Want a Pelvic Exam. She Received One Anyway" in which she explored an especially dark practice of teaching hospitals. She argues that teaching hospitals routinely train medical students on patients without obtaining their consent. Goldberg goes on to tell stories of women who specifically said they did not want to be treated by students but who woke from anesthesia and found that students had given them pelvic exams or other invasive medical testing. While sometimes students are trained to do treatments that are necessary for patients, often they are done completely for the benefit of students, without patient consent. Goldberg cites a 2005 study conducted by Stephanie Schniederjan and G. Kevin Donovan in which students reported that they believed that nearly 75 percent of the women they had given pelvic exams to had not consented to the procedure.[34] Most women who suffer from the specific mistreatment of nonconsensual gynecological exams are disproportionately low income and without insurance, the very patients most likely to rely on teaching hospitals for care.[35] Even within the hospitals, people without insurance are more likely to receive nonconsensual exams than are women with insurance.[36]

Obstetric violence still happens and, though underreported, it has gained increasing attention in news stories and academic research. This change is largely due to the attention that women in Latin America have brought to the issue.[37] Stories have appeared in such places as *Glamour* Magazine and *The Guardian* on the phenomenon of coerced cesarean.[38] The Washington Post, CNN, and other news outlets have begun reporting on obstetric violence more broadly, particularly after Evelyn Yang, whose husband Andrew Yang was a democratic candidate for president in 2020, disclosed that she had experienced such violence in childbirth.[39]

Notably absent is scholarship in law journals about the issue of obstetric violence. Those that do exist focus primarily on laws that exist outside of the United States.[40] In 2007, Venezuela passed the first law regarding obstetric violence.[41] Currently, five Latin American nations have such laws: Venezuela, Argentina, Bolivia, Panama, and Mexico.[42]

The level at which obstetric violence occurs is difficult to assess. As mentioned, women often do not report these experiences. Medical staff often remain silent as well, either for fear of retribution or because these actions have become accepted practices in their hospital or clinic's culture. Despite laws that require informed consent, as these surveys and studies show, obstetric violence continues to be a part of the childbirth experience for many women in the United States, particularly women of color, immigrants, and low-income women. I turn now to an exploration of how these practices persist, given the existing laws on informed consent.

CAUSES OF CONTEMPORARY OBSTETRIC VIOLENCE

The ability for women to have some control over their experience and as much body autonomy as possible in childbirth has profound implications for their relationship to the event. Even when birth experiences do not end up unfolding in the manner women hoped at the outset, women who feel they had choice and control in the experience feel more positive about their deliveries than do women who did not have choice or control.[43] Official organizations even advocate for women's autonomy in decisions related to childbirth. For example, the American College of Obstetrics and Gynecology Committee Opinion on Maternal Decision Making, Ethics, and the Law recommends that mothers should "not be punished for adverse perinatal outcomes" and that their "autonomous decisions should be respected."[44]

Given the vitality of mutually agreed upon care, one may question why and how non-consensual procedures persist with such frequency in obstetric medicine. This violence toward women is lurking in the invisible ways our society accepts unrelenting control over women's bodies. While most medical practitioners are unlikely to be knowingly targeting women as victims of state control, cultural stories of white supremacy, class-based oppression, and misogyny reside deep within our national knowledge. Thus, we are unable to see how the ideologies of white supremacy and misogyny shape our belief structures, our values, and the way we treat people in the world. It is in this invisibility that systems of power find their strength.

Medical practitioners, like all of us, live in a social structure, shaped by power-knowledge systems that support certain sets of interactions with patients over others. These invisible value structures underly more overt belief structures and operate in ways that trump the laws that now "require" informed consent. For example, in medical school, doctors are taught that they are to "do no harm" and "do what is best" for the patients. Yet, in making these decisions about what is best, they are also agents of broader cultural ideologies that devalue women and women's control of their bodies (and, in this case, deeply value the fetus). This lesson presents further challenge for obstetricians who are charged with caring for two patients at once. This tension is termed the maternal-fetal conflict and typically results when the needs of the two patients (mother and fetus) differ. The maternal-fetal conflict has emerged in scholarship and the practice of medicine alongside technological advances that allow doctors to better monitor the fetus during childbirth. In doing so, they have a better sense of how the fetus is doing and may press for more risky procedures for the mother to improve outcomes for infants.[45] To illustrate a situation in which this conflict is apparent, imagine that a fetus' heart rate appears to drop on the fetal monitor during labor. While this may not indicate a problem and, in the past a doctor would not have known it even occurred, in the present it is likely to cause an obstetrician to perceive the fetus as in distress and encourage a cesarean section. In doing so, the mother is placed at increased risk as cesareans are major surgeries with complications, such as infection, hemorrhage, blood clots, and other injuries.[46]

Given that to treat the fetus, a doctor must use a mother's body for access, this presents an ethical challenge when women do not consent to treatments that would benefit their baby.[47] Such a barrier also presents legal challenges for doctors who may fear repercussions in the form of malpractice suits if patient outcomes are poor (i.e., a baby dies). As a result, they may coerce or push a woman into a certain course of care.[48] Malpractice suits are most commonly brought because of infant injury or death, often because doctors did not perform a cesarean or did so too late.[49] These suits incentivize doctors to seek cesareans early in a woman's labor and more frequently than is necessary. Over 63 percent of obstetricians have been sued in their careers, the second highest rate in medicine behind surgeons.[50] Such practices likely reflect both the societal value of a baby's survival during birth and the cost associated with birth as a result of the private insurance system.

In some instances, practitioners may feel so motivated to do what they feel is best that they take for granted that their patients will agree with their course of action.[51] This assumes that patients share the moral values and hope for the same outcomes as practitioners and is, quite frankly, a dismissal of a women's agency. For example, let's imagine that a mother is suffering from a hemorrhage and will die without a blood transfusion. A doctor might not consider a situation in which she would decline this intervention and proceed accordingly. However, for women who are Jehovah's witnesses, blood transfusions are religiously prohibited, and they may refuse treatment.[52]

An example of a woman in our study who experienced an unwanted procedure assumed appropriate by a practitioner is Phoebe. Phoebe was induced at thirty-eight weeks because her fetus' heart rate was elevated. After fifty-four hours of labor, she finally delivered her daughter. Phoebe's doctors insisted on removing her daughter using suction, which Phoebe refused. She protested: "no, I don't want that. I would rather have a c-section than to have that." Yet, despite her protests, they persisted. She recalls: "I was crying, and saying 'no, I don't want this!' and they were like, 'you push, we'll pull' . . . it was just awful." Due to Phoebe's doctor's assumption that the focus of birth is the arrival of a healthy infant, they rejected Phoebe's agency in determining how her daughter would emerge through actively denying her requests.

A second set of values further complicates obstetric practice and the maternal-fetal conflict. Despite laws regarding informed consent and the official positions of medical organizations, U.S. culture places great value on the life of the fetus. At the start of this chapter, I explained how Foucault outlines the invisible ways that moral imperatives operate to control behavior in a society. In this manner, contemporary ethics regarding women as secondary to their fetus operate invisibly (as an internal message and through social sanctioning by others) to shape women's behavior. Even during pregnancy, women's behavior is policed. Women's alcohol use, smoking, or weight are targets for surveillance and criticism both socially as well as legally, wherein pregnant women have been arrested and convicted for substance abuse.[53] Courts have demanded that women undergo treatment for drug use, even against their will. They have also ordered women to undergo certain treatments or medications even if they refuse them.[54]

Advocates of this approach suggest that women in childbirth are not wholly autonomous, and thus doctors have an ethical right and duty to do what is best for the fetus.[55] Despite these sentiments, fetuses do not have legal personhood in the United States, and medical doctors do not have legal or moral power to override a woman's decision regarding her labor.[56] Yet, as is often the case, women are coerced into practices that doctors see as benefiting the fetus at risk to the mother.[57]

Cultural values produce the maternal-fetal conflict in this context. As a result of this tension, doctors often feel the need to pressure clients into consenting to certain treatments they see as advantageous to the baby. Sometimes the coercion doctors use to elicit consent is direct. Other times it is hidden or subtle. For example, doctors may exaggerate certain risks or benefits to influence a woman's decision. They may suggest a woman is a bad mother for choosing to put their fetus at risk; in some cases, even threatening to call child protective services or to remove their child upon its birth. Finally, doctors may refuse to continue working with a patient to encourage her to choose a certain course of care.[58]

To illustrate this tension more clearly, I would like to share the story of Renee. When Renee was in the hospital to deliver her daughter Sandra, her doctor recommended that she have a caesarian section. Renee's initial response was that they were "jumping the gun." She had not been in labor that long and the baby was doing well, according to the monitors. Her doctor, Dr. Spencer, told her that a "room full of OB doctors . . . almost all of them would say they wanted to deliver with a c-section." She went on to tell Renee that having a cesarean was "no big deal and that [she] should not worry about it." When this approach failed to convince Renee, Dr. Spencer told her that, if she did not have a cesarean, she would be forcing her "baby to take the risk." Renee still does not know what risks her fetus would be under, "No one ever talked to me about those risks." Despite never explaining any existing danger to Sandra, Dr. Spencer used several coercive and unethical practices to pressure Renee into a cesarean. She first minimized the risks of the cesarean. She exaggerated the dangers of waiting. She made Renee feel like a bad mother if she chose to continue vaginal delivery.

Renee also struggled with what she felt was greater care for her infant than herself throughout her delivery. She recalls that "the baby is the main focus of everything" and that "a common thing" was to do what was best for the baby. Through this process, Renee felt reduced to an object. She recalls "I felt, at this point, like I was no longer a human being. I was just this packaging for a baby that was inside of me. And you would have to rip away the packaging to get this beautiful baby on the inside. And I'm just the part that you throw away." During her daughter's birth, Renee felt discardable and unimportant as her doctors and partner placed greater value on the fetus' experience than her own. Her feeling of unimportance was especially pronounced because her doctor failed to give her any indication that doing what was best for her, and waiting for a natural start to labor, would be harmful to her daughter. Rather, they pressed the low risks of the cesarean until she acquiesced.

Beyond social standards that value fetuses at the expense of mothers, additional cultural values regarding women's (particularly poor women's) worth (or value as an object) are also at play, especially at teaching hospitals. Coldicott et al. (2003) argue that these practices are rooted in a utilitarian value system employed by such hospitals wherein "harm to one individual (the patient) may be sanctioned if it is for the benefit of a larger group (other patients)." By this logic, foregoing consent on one patient, under the guise of teaching a future doctor the procedure, is acceptable to those participating in the system.[59]

As offensive as it is, some doctors argue that patients imply consent by seeking care at a teaching hospital, others argue that patients will refuse to consent and therefore it should not be sought, while still others believe that people on Medicare in particular "owe it" to the hospital and broader society in exchange for their care.[60] Robin Wilson, law professor at the University of Illinois, in her article "Autonomy Suspended: Using Female Patients to Teach Intimate Exams Without Their Knowledge or Consent," asserts that all of these contentions are undoubtedly unfounded. People are typically unaware they are in a teaching hospital at all, much less that being there may imply consent to certain procedures. Patients often report that they would consent to certain treatments, and hospitals are adequately compensated for seeing patients without insurance.[61] Regardless of the falsehood of these claims, performing examinations on people without consent is unethical.

STRUCTURAL AND LEGAL FORCES

The power-knowledge that gave rise to the eugenics movement's value system contributed to the construction of the structural and legal forces at play that impair women's ability to consent to treatments. Many hospitals in rural communities, including North and South Hospitals, do not allow women to have vaginal births following cesareans. Though not intentionally coercive, forcing women to have a cesarean or turning her away is violating a woman's right to consent.[62] For the women in our sample, those who decide they want to have a vaginal birth following a cesarean (VBAC) are forced to seek care out of town. The closest hospital that allows VBACs is approximately 30–45 miles away. Local doctors do not practice there, so women must seek care by traveling a great distance or forego prenatal care altogether. Here we see yet another example of how space is used as a tool of control.

North and South Hospitals are not alone in these policies. Rural hospitals are far less likely than other hospitals to allow VBACs. This discrepancy is in part due to the lower rates of obstetric care in general and also a result of the ability of hospitals to provide adequate care in the event of an emergency during labor (such as having a dedicated operating room for obstetrics). In 2010, over 90 percent of women who had a cesarean delivered their subsequent children via cesarean as well. The National Institutes of Health aimed to reduce that number to 81.7 percent by 2020. As of 2018, the number had reduced to 86.7 percent.[63]

Furthermore, the legal enforcement of consent in obstetrics is lacking. Despite laws regarding informed consent, their acceptance and practice in obstetrics remain under-implemented. One cause for this is the earlier mentioned cultural perspective that women should make personal sacrifices for their fetuses and infants. Courts may believe that women who bring suit over their birth experiences are self-interested, and therefore unsympathetic.[64] Furthermore, courts often fail to recognize the trauma women may experience because of obstetric violence. This is especially true for routine treatments, such as cesareans or episiotomies.[65] Tort law requires that one is able to prove they suffered injury.[66]

Women have a difficult time proving and prosecuting obstetric violence. Lawyers rarely agree to take up these cases, except in situations with clear injury to infants. When they do undertake cases, they are often quite expensive. Tort cases involve extensive, time-consuming research and investigation.[67] Finally, as mentioned, a disproportionate number of women who experience obstetric violence are low income and unable to afford legal action.

CONCLUSION

Contemporary obstetric violence is an artifact of historical, overt, systems of power and privilege in which the state and its actors constructed a hierarchy of reproductive value and rights. While today medical practitioners are unlikely to see themselves as agents of this system, its ideological foundation continues to shape the behavior of those who operate within it. Furthermore, this knowledge (i.e., white supremacy, meritocracy, misogyny) constructing a social hierarchy serves as the foundation for the current structures within which women deliver their babies. This leaves women with little to no power or recourse.

Earlier chapters examined how poor experiences with providers exacerbate trauma for women in childbirth. I've further explored the ways that institutional and ideological systems reproduce and create these low-quality interactions. In the next chapter, I investigate how traumatic childbirth impacts women and the role that these same ideological shadows affect women's relationships to their birth experience, children, partners, and, ultimately, to themselves.

NOTES

1. Beth Israel Lahey Health—Winchester Hospital, "Cystocele/Rectocele," Nd. Accessed October 19, 2020. https://www.winchesterhospital.org/health-library/artic le?id=100092.

2. Lamaze International, "What is obstetric violence and what if it happens to you?" July 20, 2020. Accessed October 19, 2020. https://www.lamaze.org/Gi ving-Birth-with-Confidence/GBWC-Post/what-is-obstetric-violence-and-what-if-it-h appens-to-you; Farah Diaz-Tello, "Invisible wounds: Obstetric violence in the United States," *Reproductive Health Matters* 24, no. 47 (2016): 56–64; Elizabeth Kukura, "Obstetric violence," *Geo. LJ* 106 (2017): 721.

3. Michel Foucault, *"Society Must Be Defended": Lectures at the College de France 1975–1976*, ed. Mauro Bertani and Alessandro Fontana, trans. David Macey (New York: Picador, 2003).

4. Ann Laura Stoler, *Carnal Knowledge and Imperial Power: Race and the Intimate in Colonial Rule* (Berkeley: University of California Press, 2002).

5. Angie Kennedy, "Eugenics, "degenerate girls," and social workers during the progressive era." *Affilia* 23, no. 1 (2008): 22–37.

6. Kennedy, "Eugenics"; Michael G. Silver, "Eugenics and compulsory steriliza- tion laws: Providing redress for the victims of a shameful era in United States his- tory," *George Washington Law Review* 72, no. 4 (April 2004): 862–892.

7. Silver, "Eugenics and Compulsory Sterilization Laws."

8. Catherine Shoichet, "ICE hysterectomy allegations evoke US history of forced sterilizations," *CNN.* September 16, 2020. https://www.msn.com/en-us/news/us/ice -hysterectomy-allegations-evoke-us-history-of-forced-sterilizations/ar-BB196QSE.

9. André N. Sofair and Lauris C. Kaldjian, "Eugenic sterilization and a quali- fied Nazi analogy: the United States and Germany, 1930-1945," *Annals of Internal Medicine* 132, no. 4 (2000): 312–319.

10. Kennedy, "Eugenics."

11. Buck v. Bell, Superintendent of State Colony Epileptics and Feeble Minded. 274 U.S. 200. 1927. https://www.law.cornell.edu/supremecourt/text/274/200.

12. Burke Shartel, "Sterilization of mental defectives," *Journal of Criminal Law & Criminology* 16 (1925): 537.

13. Andrea Smith, *Conquest* (Boston, MA: South End Press, 2005).

14. Smith, *Conquest.*

15. Laura Briggs, *Reproducing Empire* (Berkeley, CA: University of California Press, 2001); Renee Tajima-Peña, *No Más Bebés.* 2015; Kathryn Krase, "The history of forced sterilization in the United States," *Our Bodies Ourselves.* October 1, 2014. Accessed October 19, 2020. https://www.ourbodiesourselves.org/book-excerpts/h ealth-article/forced-sterilization/.

16. Tom L. Beauchamp, "Informed consent: Its history, meaning, and present challenges," *Cambridge Quarterly of Healthcare Ethics* 20, no. 4 (2011): 515–523; Hindi Stohl, "Childbirth is not a medical emergency: Maternal right to informed con- sent throughout labor and delivery," *Journal of Legal Medicine* 38, no. 3–4 (2018): 329–353.

17. Beauchamp, "Informed Consent"; *Canterbury v. Spence,* 464 F.2d 772 (D.C. Curcuit 1972); Stohl, "Childbirth is not a medical emergency."

18. Beauchamp, "Informed Consent."

19. Beauchamp, "Informed Consent."

20. MCN, *The American Journal of Maternal/Child Nursing* 2, no. 2 (March–April 1977): 137–138.

21. Andrew Almand, "A mother's worst nightmare, what's left unsaid," *William and Mary Journal of Race, Gender, and Social Justice* 18, no. 3 (2012).

22. David M. Studdert, Michelle M. Mello, Marin K. Levy, Russell L. Gruen, Edward J. Dunn, E. John Orav, and Troyen A. Brennan, "Geographic variation in informed consent law: Two standards for disclosure of treatment risks," *Journal of Empirical Legal Studies* 4, no. 1 (2007): 103–124.

23. American Medical Association, "Informed Consent," Accessed February 5, 2021. https://www.ama-assn.org/delivering-care/ethics/informed-consent.

24. Lamaze International, "What is obstetric violence and what if it happens to you?" July 20, 2020. Accessed October 19, 2020. https://www.lamaze.org/Giving-Birth-with-Confidence/GBWC-Post/what-is-obstetric-violence-and-what-if-it-happens-to-you; Elizabeth Kukura, "Obstetric violence," *Georgetown Law Journal* 106 (2017): 721.

25. Rebecca Schiller, *Why Human Rights in Childbirth Matter* (London: Pinter and Martin, 2017).

26. Kukura, "Obstetric violence," 721.

27. Lisa Ko, "Unwanted sterilization and eugenics programs in the United States," *Independent Lens.* January 29, 2016. Accessed October 10, 2020. https://www.pbs.org/independentlens/blog/unwanted-sterilization-and-eugenics-programs-in-the-united-states/; Shilpa Jindia, "Belly of the Beast: California's dark history of forced sterilizations," *The Guardian.* June 30, 2020. Accessed October 1, 2020. https://www.theguardian.com/us-news/2020/jun/30/california-prisons-forced-sterilizations-belly-beast.

28. Shilpa. "Belly of the Beast."

29. Erika Cohn, 2020. *Belly of the Beast.*

30. Shilpa. "Belly of the Beast."

31. Rachel Treisman, "Whistleblower alleges 'medical neglect,' questionable hysterectomies of ICE detainees," September 16, 2020. Accessed October 5, 2020. https://www.wbez.org/stories/whistleblower-alleges-medical-neglect-questionable-hysterectomies-of-ice-detainees/e5b12292-62d4-4df7-b12e-cc650e3f07d7.

32. Treisman, 2020, "Whistleblower Alleges 'Medical Neglect.'"

33. Louise Marie Roth, Nicole Heidbreder, Megan M. Henley, Marla, Marek, Miriam Naiman-Sessions, Jennifer, Torres, and Christine H. Morton, "Maternity support survey: A report on the criss-national surveys of Doulas, Childbirth Educators and labor and delivery nurses in the United States and Canada." May 1, 2014. Accessed September 29, 2020. https://maternitysurvey.files.wordpress.com/2014/07/mss-report-5-1-14-final.pdf.

34. Stephanie Schniederjan and G. Kevin Donovan, "Ethics versus education: Pelvic exams on anesthetized women," *The Journal of the Oklahoma State Medical Association* 98, no. 8 (2005): 386–388.

35. Robin Fretwell Wilson, "Autonomy suspended: Using female patients to teach intimate exams without their knowledge or consent," *Journal of Health Care Law & Policy* 8, no. 2, 2005, 240–263.

36. Wilson, "Autonomy Suspended," 240–263.

37. Kukura, "Obstetric violence," 721.

38. Molly Redden, "New York hospital's secret policy led to woman being given c-section against her will," *The Guardian.* October 5, 2017. Accessed September 30, 2020. https://www.theguardian.com/us-news/2017/oct/05/new-york-staten-island-university-hospital-c-section-ethics-medicine; https://www.glamour.com/story/new-moms-c-sections-without-consent.

39. Kimberley Seals Allers, "Obstetric violence is a real problem. Evelyn Yang's experience is just one example," *The Washington Post.* February 6, 2020. Accessed October 20, 2020. https://www.washingtonpost.com/lifestyle/2020/02/06/obstetric-violence-is-real-problem-evelyn-yangs-experience-is-just-one-example/; Robert Kuznia, Nelli Black, and Drew Griffin, "Evelyn Yang says Columbia University and New York DA 'grossly mishandled' case of OB-GYN she accuses of sexual assault," *CNN.* February 21, 2020. Accessed October 18, 2020. https://www.cnn.com/2020/02/21/politics/evelyn-yang-marissa-hoechstetter-vance-invs/index.html.

40. Kukura, "Obstetric violence," 721.

41. Caitlin R. Williams, Celeste Jerez, Karen Klein, Malena Correa, Jose Belizan, and Gabriela Cormick, "Obstetric violence: A Latin American legal response to mistreatment during childbirth," *An International Journal of Obstetrics and Gynaecology* 125, no. 10 (2018): 1208–1211.

42. Williams et al., "Obstetric violence," 1208–1211.

43. Katie Cook and Collen Loomis, "The impact of choice and control on women's childbirth experiences," *Journal of Perinatal Education* 21, no. 3 (2012): 158–168.

44. Susan F. Townsend, "Obstetric conflict: When fetal and maternal interests are at odds," *Pediatrics in Review* 32, no. 1 (2012): 33–36; American College of Obstetricians and Gynecologists, "Ethical decision making in obstetrics and gynecology," Committee Opinion No. 390, December 2007. Accessed October 20, 2020. http://www.acog.org/from_home/ publications/ethics/co390.pdf.

45. Townsend, "Obstetric conflict," 33–36.

46. The Mayo Clinic, "C-section." Accessed November 21, 2020. https://www.mayoclinic.org/tests-procedures/c-section/about/pac-20393655.

47. Townsend, "Obstetric conflict," 33–36.

48. Andrew Kotaska, "Informed consent and refusal in obstetrics: A practical ethical guide," *Birth* 44, no. 3 (2017): 195–199.

49. Andrea M. Carpentieri, James J. Lumalcuri, Jennie Shaw, and G. F. Joseph, "Overview of the 2015 American Congress of Obstetricians and Gynecologists' survey on professional liability," *Clinical Review* 20 (2015): 1–6.

50. José Guardado, "Medical liability claims frequency among U.S. physicians," *American Medical Association.* Accessed November 21, 2020. https://www.ama-assn.org/practice-management/sustainability/medical-liability-market-research.

51. Kotaska, "Informed consent and refusal in obstetrics," 195–199.

52. Kotaska, "Informed consent and refusal in obstetrics," 195–199.

53. Rebecca Stone, "Pregnant women and substance use: Fear, stigma, and barriers to care," *Health Justice* 3, no 2 (2015).

54. Lisa Cosgrove and Akansha Vaswani, "Fetal rights, the policing of pregnancy, and meanings of the maternal in an age of neoliberalism," *Journal of Theoretical and Philosophical Psychology* 40, no. 1 (2020): 43.

55. Kotaska, "Informed consent and refusal in obstetrics," 195–199.

56. Kotaska, "Informed consent and refusal in obstetrics," 195–199.

57. Susan S Mattingly, "The maternal–fetal dyad exploring the two-patient obstetric model," *The Hastings Center Report* 22, no. 1 (1992): 13–18. Accessed October 16, 2020. doi:10.2307/3562716.

58. Kotaska, "Informed consent and refusal in obstetrics," 195–199.

59. Yvette Coldicott, Britt-Ingjerd Nesheim, Jane MacDougall, Catherine Pope, and Clive Roberts, "The ethics of intimate examinations—Teaching tomorrow's doctorsCommentary: Respecting the patient's integrity is the keyCommentary: Teaching pelvic examination—Putting the patient first," *Bmj* 326, no. 7380 (2003): 97–101.

60. Jude T. Waterbury, "Refuting patients' obligations to clinical training: a critical analysis of the arguments for an obligation of patients to participate in the clinical education of medical students." *Medical Education* 35, no. 3 (2001): 286–294; Wilson, "Autonomy Suspended," 240–263.

61. Wilson, "Autonomy Suspended," 240–263.

62. Kotaska, "Informed consent and refusal in obstetrics," 195–199.

63. Cesarean Rates, "Understanding cesarean rates," Accessed September 25, 2020. https://www.cesareanrates.org; Martin, Joyce A., Brady E. Hamilton, Michelle J. K. Osterman, Sally C. Curtin, and T. J. Mathews, "Births: Final data for 2013 (National Vital Statistics Reports, Vol. 64, No. 1)," *Hyattsville, MD: National Center for Health Statistics* (2015); Osterman, Michelle JK, and Joyce A. Martin. "Trends in low-risk cesarean delivery in the United States, 1990–2013." (2014).

64. Kukura, "Obstetric violence," 721.

65. Kukura, "Obstetric violence," 721.

66. Kukura, "Obstetric violence," 721.

67. Kukura, "Obstetric violence," 721.

Chapter 5

"We Perpetuate the Patriarchy"

The Trauma Imposed by Societal Knowledge

Alice's dream of the perfect birth began early in her life. An Anthropology major in college, her idealizing of a so-called "natural birth" grew expansively. In her words, "I wanted this labor. I had this beautiful pregnancy and I wanted to be a participant in evolution." She had even written "be a participant in evolution" in her birth plan. She continued, "I wanted to be my animal self and I didn't get that . . . that's my biggest disappointment."

Instead, following about thirty hours of labor, Alice started to become dehydrated and weak from vomiting. Her midwife encouraged her to transfer from the birth center to the hospital to get an epidural. She did. But, after the intervention, nurses realized that her baby's heart rate was not responding appropriately to contractions. They kept an eye on the baby while Alice spent the next few hours pushing. Not making any progress, her baby's heart rate continued to climb, and her doctor notified her "we're at a point where we need to do a c-section." Alice felt "totally" blindsided.

Alice's explanation of her disappointment deepened as she shared that her inability to naturally deliver her child makes her feel like a failure, "People have done this forever. It is the point of existence. I should be able to . . . What is it about me that makes it so that I shouldn't be able to do that?" She reflected on women throughout history and her love of the TV show *Call the Midwife* and her eyes sharpened. In that moment she realized that, if she had needed to deliver her baby a century earlier, "maybe I would have died."

In our interviews, the women we talked to struggled extensively with their mental health following the delivery of their child. They experienced anxiety, postpartum depression, flashbacks, nightmares, and memory loss—all common symptoms for trauma survivors. In addition to these battles, they also faced struggles produced through the internalization of societal knowledge; they wrestle with self-blame, a sense of alienation from other mothers, and the belief that they failed. While the degree to which depression, anxiety, and flashbacks may be innate or socially influenced is hard to tease apart, the perception that one who does not have a "typical" birth is to blame or is a failure as a mother is a cultural story.

In this chapter, I look at the impact birth trauma has on the women who survive it. I'll briefly showcase the psychological struggles faced by women and how they manifest, before turning to those that are more decisively socially shaped. Foucault contends that the success of biopower is in its subtly: not only in how it operates through structures but also how it is internalized by its subjects. These systems of power shape societal norms, control people's thoughts, and impact behavior. With these processes in mind, I return to look at how ideologies and structures (power-knowledge) are reproduced even by those they hurt. To do this, I draw on both existing literature on American culture regarding childbirth and women's stories to show how the American pressure to have a (culturally defined) "ideal" birth injures women who are unable to do so.

IMPACT OF DIFFICULT CHILDBIRTH
ON MATERNAL MENTAL HEALTH

It may seem logical or be commonly assumed that the psychological reactions to traumatic events are hardwired. In truth, most responses to extreme stress are significantly shaped by societal norms and values (power-knowledge). These norms and values impact whether or not someone seeks mental health care, what types of intervention they consider, strategies they have to manage mental health challenges, and the nature of their support networks.[1] There is also evidence that the very symptoms people experience are influenced by societal expectations.[2] This is evidence of the way that power-knowledge shapes the way people behave and, even, how they think and feel.

For example, doctors and researchers Hoang and Erickson; Lin, Carter, and Kleinman; and Mollica find that in certain Southeastern Asian cultures, trauma often manifests as head pain. This is explained at least partially by cultural prioritization of the head as especially valued.[3] In contrast, trauma often manifests in Latin American cultures as afflictions of the nervous system (dizziness, etc.).[4] In Europe and the United States, people who face trauma tend to have fewer somatic symptoms, but instead experience psychological challenges such as nervousness or an incapability to relax.[5] Howard Waitzkin and Holly Magaña review this literature and summarize scholarship on this issue noting that, though not every individual in a society will respond to trauma identically, culture shapes how people "process their narratives of severe trauma."[6]

Relating to birth trauma specifically, social knowledge has an impact on the prevalence and manifestation of trauma. In places where mothers are provided greater postpartum support and care, women's experiences of postpartum depression are moderated (unless that care is poorly provided).[7] Social norms can also shape how women manage their struggles. In her dissertation, Professor Linda Amankwaa, nursing faculty at Albany State University, found that Black women felt pressure to be "strong" and that suffering from postnatal depression was something only white women were permitted to do. Instead, Amankwaa argues, Black women are more likely to turn to religious communities for support. Furthermore, Tanya Paul, a registered nurse at Connecticut Children's Hospital, finds that culture may play a role in how one responds to postnatal PTSD. In her study of difficult childbirths, trauma, and the impacts on women, Paul found that white women are more likely than Latina women to avoid thoughts or activities in response to experiencing trauma.[8]

The women in our sample primarily struggled with symptoms culturally associated with postpartum depression, postpartum anxiety, and postnatal posttraumatic stress disorder. However, most women we talked with did not have access to or otherwise seek postpartum psychological care. This is not unusual. Mental health disorders, in general, are undertreated. In fact, the *Journal of the American Medical Association* reported in 2000 that as many as 50 percent of Americans with "severe mental illness" fail to seek treatment, even when it is available.[9] Data from the 2017 National Survey on Drug Use and Health suggests that these numbers remain equally bleak in the present.[10] The U.S. Surgeon General, David Satcher, proposes that people choose not to seek treatment because of the stigmas associated with mental health problems (the internalization of societal knowledge) and the cost of mental health services, among other obstacles.[11] This is especially true for new mothers who, in addition to barriers resulting from stigma and expenses, often fear involvement from child protective services (CPS) if they admit to struggling with mental illness.[12] Women of color, in particular, face a heightened risk of CPS intervention as a result of personal and structural racism, and therefore feel unable to seek mental health care following childbirth.[13]

Despite not seeking or receiving treatment, many women in our sample experienced severe, debilitating, and long-lasting symptoms of depression. Postpartum depression affects around 15 percent of new mothers.[14] It is distinct from what has been referred to as the "baby blues" and is characterized by a "depressed mood or loss of interest or pleasure in activities" lasting for more than two weeks.[15] People who have cesarean sections or a negative birth experience have an elevated risk of experiencing postpartum depression.[16]

One woman in our sample, Lisa, who was transferred while pregnant to a regional urban hospital due to severe preeclampsia, continued to struggle with extreme sadness at our interview months later. She recalled how people frequently remind her that she has "a healthy baby." This not only serves to inadvertently dismiss her experience, but it also furthers her guilt for continuing to struggle herself. Lisa assured me that she is "really grateful for that" but that she also knows "he doesn't have a healthy mom and that's really hard. It's really hard, wishing on a daily basis that . . . had things gone differently that day, maybe he would've been better off. Maybe he would have a chance at a happier childhood cause he wouldn't have a mom that's a mess every day." Pausing for a moment to reflect on the magnitude of Lisa's claim is important. Here she says her son would be better off had she died during childbirth. That's how unwell Lisa still felt months after his birth.

Lisa, like many women in our sample, had taken the routinely administered postpartum depression screenings at previous doctor's visits. While the Center for Disease Control recommends every mother be screened, they estimate that up to 13 percent of women are never asked about depression during a postnatal visit.[17] Like many women we talked with, Lisa lied on the form. She was afraid that, if she told them the truth, they'd "take my baby away from me." She told her doctor her concerns and was assured that she would feel better in three months. Even though her doctor knew she falsified the forms, Lisa was not referred for psychological or even additional medical postpartum care.

Lisa and other women's fear that they may have their babies removed from their homes, is indicative of the power-knowledge system at play in this instance. In his work, *Discipline and Punish*, Foucault not only explores how time, space, and routine are employed to exert state control. He further examines the use of surveillance. In discussing the Panopticon, a guard tower at a prison that allows guards to see in all directions but not be seen themselves, Foucault analyzes the power of feared surveillance. Foucault contends that a guard need never be in the tower for it to have the effect of controlling prisoner actions; simply the possibility that a guard may be watching is enough to influence behavior.[18] In Lisa's case, we see how the fear of CPS operates in the same way. Women are afraid to disclose their mental health challenges to their doctors and their behavior is moderated, simply based on the possible threat this surveillance poses.

Postpartum anxiety (PPA) is not officially listed in the DSM as a standalone condition and is often regarded as a symptom of postpartum depression, an associated mood disorder, or even a form of generalized anxiety disorder (GAD). PPA affects around 17 percent of new mothers.[19] As with postpartum depression, the experience of a difficult childbirth increases a mother's likelihood of struggling with PPA following the baby's birth.

Many women in our sample experienced heightened anxiety following their child's birth. For example, Beth describes how worrying led her to lose significant sleep. Beth had an emergency cesarean following a transfer from the birth center to the hospital, because the baby was "a surprise breech." After this experience, she wrestled with extreme anxiety, "I've been having some issues with insomnia . . . . I've always been a little bit of a worry-wort but now it's more like, let's take it to an extreme. Like, 'what if she pulls the cover up over her head and suffocates? Instead of being like 'that's not going to happen'. . . I definitely make it a little more extreme, and I'm pretty sure that's kind of a posttraumatic kind of thing."

Participants also wrestled with intrusive thoughts; another symptom commonly associated with postpartum depression. One woman in our sample, Amber, faced this burden. During her scheduled cesarean, Amber experienced failed anesthesia. Her doctor did not believe her, and she went through the surgery experiencing extreme pain. When she got home from the hospital, she could not fight the intrusive thoughts that kept replying in her mind. Amber recalls, "After she was born all I could think about was hurting her. I didn't want to think about it, but I couldn't control it. It was all I could think about." Intrusive thoughts such as Amber's are often considered to be a manifestation of obsessive-compulsive disorder associated with postpartum depression.

In addition to depression and anxiety, the women we talked to also experienced other symptoms of trauma including flashbacks and nightmares. Natalie's baby was born six weeks premature after she went into early labor and was sent via air ambulance to an urban hospital with a NICU. He then spent nearly four weeks in the NICU before the family was able to return home. When she finally got back to her hometown, Natalie began to experience extreme insomnia as a result of flashbacks, "I remember getting so frustrated when it'd be in the middle of the night and he'd be asleep and I could not sleep, I was just like, thinking, just replaying everything, and how things could've gone worse, and I just could not stop thinking." Flashbacks are a common symptom of postpartum posttraumatic stress disorder along with nightmares, avoidance, and nervous system arousal.[20]

Few of the women we talked to were officially diagnosed with any mental disorders during or following childbirth, though they clearly experienced severe symptoms associated with depression, anxiety, and posttraumatic stress disorder. In truth, mental health disorders associated with childbirth are underdiagnosed.[21] As I outline the experiences of women here, I do not seek to offer a diagnosis for our participants. Rather, I aim to explain how culture shapes both the response to trauma and difficult childbirths as well as the way cultural norms and expectations around birth cause harm to women, which I turn to now.

THE GENEALOGY OF "IDEAL BIRTH"

Beyond commonly understood mental health struggles, such as depression, anxiety, and posttraumatic stress disorder, the women in our sample suffered as a result of their inability to perform what they internalized as an ideal birth. These norms around childbirth left mothers wounded, first by the trauma of a near loss of life and then, again, by societal knowledge that devalues their experience. Through internalizing these norms, women self-sanction—punish, surveille, or blame themselves for the problems faced during childbirth. They view themselves as a failure and experience associated emotions of guilt and shame. It also causes women to feel alienated from other mothers and, for some, even from themselves. The women we talked to expressed feeling a severe sense of loss by not being able to meet cultural standards regarding birth.

In chapter 3, I traced the genealogy of the modern obstetric care system in the United States. I explained how the 1800s were a period of homebirth in which births were a social affair for women. Births were attended by friends, family, and a midwife. Fear of pain associated with childbirth and concurrent medical advances led to the medicalization of childbirth at the turn of the century. Midwives were replaced by doctors, who were exclusively men. The cesarean rate exploded. Women began to feel disconnected from childbirth. In response, a new cultural movement, the natural birth movement, arose critiquing the medicalization of childbirth. Parallel to these changes was the evolution of societal knowledge surrounding the cesarean.

The cesarean as performed on a living woman, who survived, was first accomplished around 1820. It was conducted by Dr. James Miranda Stuart Barry, a physician and woman, who had to disguise herself as a man to practice medicine.[22] Prior to this time, there is some evidence that cesareans were performed in ancient Greece, though on deceased or dying mothers. Though in rare circumstances it seems that women survived, the cesarean did not aim to preserve a woman's life.[23]

Until the 1850s, cesareans were performed without anesthesia.[24] At first, this was because it had not been developed for medical use, but later in European and American societies, because Christian-influenced cultural norms touted that childbirth should be painful as punishment for Eve's original sin.[25] Unfortunately, this belief has not fully disappeared from people's belief structures, including those of some obstetricians.[26]

I want to emphasize this example. Medical practitioners did not use anesthesia on women in childbirth, even those having cesareans, because social knowledge dictated that they should suffer during childbirth. Though just one instance, this is a clear example of how cultural norms (in this case, religious-based misogyny) cause trauma.

By the mid-1900s, anesthesia had improved and the number of women having cesareans increased dramatically. About 32 percent of babies currently born in the United States are delivered via cesarean, an increase of 20 percent since 1970.[27] This rise aligns with advances in technology that monitor fetuses in utero, including the fetal heart monitor (itself critiqued as one of the most commonly employed intervention administered without a mother's informed consent).[28] It also runs parallel to a cultural shift placing the baby, and not the mother, as the central patient during childbirth.[29] This increase in cesarean rates has largely been in response to a rise in caution with regard to the well-being of babies during delivery. Cesarean rates are especially high in rural communities among mothers of all races and among Black, Latinx, and Native American women in other regions. There is also a strong association between level of education and cesarean rate, suggesting that poor-quality maternal care results in higher cesarean rates for vulnerable populations.[30] Cesarean rates also vary significantly by hospital and even physician.[31]

Despite, or perhaps because, the United States has an unusually high number of caesarian sections, it is also home to specific cultural backlash against cesarean use. Celebrities such as Ricki Lake are well known for their opposition to elective cesareans specifically. In 2008, Ricki Lake and Abby Epstein directed a film called *The Business of Being Born* within which Lake is featured having a home birth with her first child, Owen. While in the film Lake states that she believes people can feel empowered via elective cesarean, the directors go on to argue that cesareans are overperformed for the convenience of the doctor and the financial benefits to the hospital of the procedure. They advocate that cesareans should be reserved for use only when the child or mother is in distress. Yet, the participants in our study who watched the film also felt it implied that a "natural" birth was superior to any involving intervention and especially the cesareans. The directors went on to make a sequel in 2011 echoing these themes and further critiquing the medicalization of childbirth.

Even people who have had cesareans malign them in the public eye. Kate Hudson, an actress, famously remarked that giving birth via cesarean was the "laziest thing [she had] ever done" on a survey given to her by *Cosmopolitan* magazine.[32] Newspaper headlines also perpetuate the idea that cesareans are the "easy" way to deliver babies. For example, the Orlando Sentinel ran a story called "Celebrity C-sections: Guess Who's Too Posh to Push" implying that cesareans are the elite way to give birth.[33] Yet other celebrities feel shame around their cesareans. For example, Kate Winslet famously lied about delivering her first-born baby, Mia, "naturally" when she actually had an emergency cesarean. She told reporters that she initially lied because failing to deliver vaginally left her feeling like a "failure."[34]

The World Health Organization puts the "acceptable rate" of cesareans around 5–15 percent while a recent study by surgeon and researcher George Molina and colleagues, in the *Journal of the American Medical Association*, puts it closer to 19 percent.[35] This indicates that cesareans are used in the United States more often than they are needed. Certainly, decreasing their use when not necessary to save babies or mothers would reduce the trauma experienced by women in childbirth. Yet, of interest in this chapter is the way that cultural norms in certain communities around the superiority of "natural births" are instrumental in the traumatization of mothers who deliver via cesarean. Below I explore the subcultural norms that influenced the mothers in our sample and how their inability to meet these expectations harmed women.

HOW INTERNALIZED POWER-KNOWLEDGE HARMS MOTHERS

There is not a single U.S. culture surrounding childbirth. Rather, there are class, racial, age, and geographic differences in social stories regarding what is a "good" birth. While middle-class women often seek to control the events of their birth (i.e., what sorts of treatment they experience), working-class women are more likely to value governing their pain levels and personal behavior instead.[36] The women in our sample by and large subscribed to the cultural script regarding the superiority of "natural birth." Their inability to achieve this goal, then, caused them additional pain beyond the psychological effects of difficult labor.

We asked the women we interviewed what they envisioned for their birth and how they came to that perspective. Most of our participants anticipated having a "natural" birth—one they defined as without intervention, indicating a strong subculture valuing childbirth such births. Some women hoped to deliver at home, others at a birth center with a midwife, and still others at the hospital. For example, Ashley recalls wanting to have an intervention-free birth in the hospital, "I wanted to just have a natural birth without any sort of intervention, like drugs." When we asked her where this image came from, she recalled several places that shaped her vision: her birthing class on the Bradley method, several books she read, an audio CD about hypnobirthing, information from La Leche League, and the aforementioned film by Lake and Epstein. The most powerful force in shaping her vision, though, was her mother. Ashley explains, "My mom was very much—I mean, she had all of my brothers and I in the hospital, which was fine, I was fine with the hospital birth. I just wanted it to be natural. My mom had all three of us naturally and stayed home, was very much like that whole attachment parenting sort of style. I think that's where my whole value and idea of what I wanted came from."

Other women just "had a sense" that unmedicated births were better than medicated births in general and superior, especially, to cesareans. They place this sentiment on images and stories they heard casually throughout their lives. For example, Hannah remembers putting together her image of the perfect birth from information she had seen as an adolescent and then later as an adult, "It probably came from magazines, and the media, and I have a really good friend that's a birthing photographer." Similarly Kayla points to "stories you hear" as the source of her interest in natural childbirth. She recalls that you never hear about "bad things" that happen until or unless you know someone personally who had difficulty. These stories are not part of the broader cultural narrative about childbirth.

Ricki Lake and Abby Epstein's film and the people featured within it were widely cited by women in our sample as a factor in shaping their thoughts regarding childbirth. In addition to Ashley above, Natalie said that the main force in shaping her views on ideal childbirth was the midwife featured in the film, Ina May. Natalie says,

> She's my whole upbringing . . . My mom is a nurse . . . for the majority of her career she was an OB nurse, or a nurse manager managing OB nurses. So, I grew up around birth. And my mom, one of her proudest accomplishments was that she had a VBAC with me . . . And she's very feministy in her own way, in this very birth is a natural process, not something that needs to be medicated and you know. She gave me Ina May's book to read, and it's all about how American women are conditioned to be afraid of childbirth and it's just a natural process . . . And also, my own feminism made me be like, I don't want to give birth to my baby on my back because women started doing that cause it was more convenient for male doctors, you know? So that's where it all started, and then working with my midwife, and my mindful birthing class, which I just really kinda honed in on what I wanted the experience to be like.

Kate Hudson, the women we interviewed, and Lake and Epstein's film point to broad elements of culture that normalize birth without interventions. Jen, who experienced a long labor followed by a cesarean due to a breeched baby, however, points to the power of this story in the local culture of Springfield, a town inhabited by a significant number of highly educated white women. She argues "I feel like a lot of it is [that] Springfield is such a natural birth community." This local culture was enriched by Jen's engagement with national media including Lake and Epstein's film, "I watched 'The Business of Being Born' and then 'More Business of Being Born' which was interesting because they did have that; they had women talking about their birth experiences and then having to have the c-section and then feeling really bad about it."

The idea that unmedicated births are "natural" made women feel as though they failed as women or even mammals in their inability to deliver vaginally. They reflected on how, in Dee's words, "People deliver babies all over the world every day." In response, the women we talked with felt shame or humiliation from not living up to cultural standards. Ashley feels like she was thrown in an unknown competition when she opted to give birth. She says, "It's almost like people feel like . . . it's this competition or something . . . I don't like it when people kind of make it like this, 'oh, I did not have any drugs.' Like a trophy or something that you get." Nancy even recalls a friend telling her that she "did not give birth because she had a c-section."

Women also struggled deeply with not feeling as though they were allowed to share their birth stories with others. For example, Beth recalls being told by her mother that "you shouldn't be telling people when they're going to have kids." She struggled because many of her friends had not yet had kids but planned to in the future. Though she wished that she had heard about people's experiences with emergency situations, her friends seemed unwilling to hear these stories. In contrast, she felt that other people she knew who also encountered unexpected events during delivery compared traumas. In Beth's words, "You either end up, like competing, like 'mine was worse than yours' competition or people are so uncomfortable that they don't really acknowledge what you say." Kathy agrees that the silence around difficult or traumatic birth hurts women. She argues, "We have to be more open to talking about hard births. We're not helping parents by hiding it."

The women we talked to felt like they failed as mothers and women in their inability to have a "perfect" childbirth. Hannah sums this up by saying, "I feel like it made me feel more like a bad mom. For some reason I am incapable of carrying a child like I should, so yeah it probably impacted my feelings as a woman and as a mother."

This sense of failure plagues women and leads them to constantly reflect on and second guess their actions during pregnancy and childbirth. For example, Alice wonders

"Like, what if I would've eaten more? Because then maybe I wouldn't have been that exhausted. Or, like, when she told me to bear down, and like, see if my water would break, I feel like maybe I kept bearing down the whole time and that's why I was swollen. So, if I hadn't had done that, or—I feel like I was not as receptive as I wished I would've been to like new positions and things like that. So, if I had done more of the things they were suggesting . . . ."

The experience of having a birth deemed atypical or unideal by one's broader culture also leaves mothers feeling alienated from other women. First, in their sense that they cannot share their stories but, second, by eliciting a feeling of jealousy or even fear toward other pregnant women. For example, Kayla mentions that she feels a sense of "envy" toward pregnant women. She shares, "I can see a pregnant woman that's, you know, holding her toddler and doing other things. Whatever, working out in the gym, like it almost makes me mad that she has this experience and I didn't." Renee believes that her feeling of disconnect is a result of local cultural stories about childbirth. She suggests, "the narrative that our society has given me about birth and delivery is that I would have this beautiful baby and I would feel connected to it and I would breastfeed, and everything would be great and those didn't happen. And so, I don't have any other narratives to compare my experience to. I feel very alone and isolated."

CONCLUSION

In his work on systems of power, Foucault argues that the success of bio-power is rooted in its ability to make power-knowledge accepted as normal such that people police their own behavior in accordance. In the case of birth trauma, we find that many of our participants speak at length about their long-seated desire for a "natural" birth. These women never even considered another option. The internalization of the knowledge that "natural" birth is superior to a cesarean or even a medicated birth caused severe psychological harm for women who were unable to attain them.

The very mental health struggles women face—postpartum depression, postpartum anxiety, and postpartum posttraumatic stress disorder—are shaped by the rules of a given society. Societies determine how, when, and where it is appropriate for women to struggle, grieve, and heal. Social norms and expectations around ideal birth further injure women who experienced difficult or traumatic childbirth. By privileging unmedicated childbirth as ideal, women who choose or need to use interventions feel as though they fail. It further hurts their sense of self, their confidence as mothers, and their relationships to other women.

While subcultures within the United States have different norms and values regarding the best way to deliver babies, the women in my sample all expressed their influence by a culture that valued unmedicated, vaginal births. As a result, women who experienced difficult and traumatic births, which in our sample exclusively required medical intervention in some way, felt as if they failed as mothers and women. The trauma they experienced which, even in absence of cultural pressures, is associated with increased rates of depression, anxiety, and posttraumatic stress disorder led many women to struggle with their mental health. The sense of failure they felt as a result of medical intervention then exacerbated this trauma. Women largely did not seek medical care for their struggles with mental health, because they feared negative repercussions.

One participant, Trish, synthesized the traumatic influence of culture on women succinctly. She argued in her interview, "We perpetuate the patriarchy in how we look at each other, and how we demand that your experience must be the same as mine or I cannot value your difference and your experience because unless it looks like mine it's not, it's not ok, right? You have to fit in my box, and that's the patriarchy."

NOTES

1. Office of the Surgeon General (US); Center for Mental Health Services (US); National Institute of Mental Health (US), "Chapter 2 Culture Counts: The Influence of Culture and Society on Mental Health," *Mental Health: Culture, Race, and Ethnicity: A Supplement to Mental Health: A Report of the Surgeon General* (Rockville, MD: Substance Abuse and Mental Health Services Administration, 2001). Available from: https://www.ncbi.nlm.nih.gov/books/NBK44249/.

2. Allan V. Horwitz, "The sociological study of mental illness," In *Handbook of the Sociology of Mental Health*, 57–78 (Boston, MA: Springer, 1999).

3. Giao N. Hoang, and Roy V. Erickson, "Guidelines for providing medical care to Southeast Asian refugees," *Jama* 248, no. 6 (1982): 710–714; E. H. Lin, William B. Carter, and Arthur M. Kleinman, "An exploration of somatization among Asian refugees and immigrants in primary care," *American Journal of Public Health* 75, no. 9 (1985): 1080–1084; Richard R. Mollica, "The trauma story: The psychiatric care of refugee survivors of violence and torture," In *Post- Traumatic Therapy and Victims of Violence*, edited by F. Ochberg, 295–314 (New York: Brunner/Mazel, 1988).

4. Ronald Angel and Peter J. Guarnaccia, "Mind, body, and culture: Somatization among Hispanics," *Social Science & Medicine* 28, no. 12 (1989): 1229–1238; Javier I. Escobar, Glorisa Canino, Maritza Rubio-Stipec, and Milagros Bravo, "Somatic symptoms after a natural disaster: A prospective study," *The American Journal of Psychiatry* (1992).

5. Elizabeth A. Hoge, Sharad M. Tamrakar, Kelly M. Christian, Namrata Mahara, Mahendra K. Nepal, Mark H. Pollack, and Naomi M. Simon, "Cross-cultural differences in somatic presentation in patients with generalized anxiety disorder." *The Journal of Nervous and Mental Disease* 194, no. 12 (2006): 962–966.

6. Howard Waitzkin and Holly Magana, "The black box in somatization: Unexplained physical symptoms, culture, and narratives of trauma." *Social Science & Medicine* 45, no. 6 (1997): 811–825.

7. Salima S. Gulamani, Shahirose Sadrudin Premji, ZeenatKhanu Kanji, and Syed Iqbal Azam, "A review of postpartum depression, preterm birth, and culture," *The Journal of Perinatal & Neonatal Nursing* 27, no. 1 (2013): 52–59.

8. Tanya A. Paul, "Prevalence of posttraumatic stress symptoms after childbirth: Does ethnicity have an impact?" *The Journal of Perinatal Education* 17, no. 3 (2008): 17–26. doi:10.1624/105812408X324534.

9. Joan Stephenson, "Mental disorders undertreated," *Jama* 283, no. 3 (2000): 325–325.

10. Substance Abuse and Mental Health Services Administration, "Key substance use and mental health indicators in the United States: Results from the 2017 National Survey on Drug Use and Health" (HHS Publication No. SMA 18-5068, NSUDH Series H-53). Rockville, MD: Center for Behavioral Health Statistics and Quality, Substance Abuse and Mental Health Services Administration. Retrieved from https://www.samhsa.gov/data/sites/default/files/cbhsq-reports/NSDUHFFR2017/NSDUHFFR2017.pdf.

11. Stephenson. "Mental Disorders Undertreated," 325.

12. Nancy Byatt, Kathleen Biebel, Liz Friedman, Gifty Debordes-Jackson, and Douglas Ziedonis, "Women's perspectives on postpartum depression screening in pediatric settings: A preliminary study," *Archives of Women's Mental Health* 16, no. 5 (2013): 429–432.

13. Aneri Pattani, "Silenced by Fear," *The Philadelphia Inquirer.* April 5, 2019. https://www.inquirer.com/health/a/postpartum-depression-perinatal-mental-health-new-mom-women-of-color-20190405.html; December Maxwell, Sarah R. Robinson, and Kelli Rogers, "I keep it to myself": A qualitative meta-interpretive synthesis of experiences of postpartum depression among marginalised women," *Health & Social Care in the Community* 27, no. 3 (2019): e23–e36.

14. Teri Pearlstein, Margaret Howard, Amy Salisbury, and Caron Zlotnick, "Postpartum depression," *American Journal of Obstetrics and Gynecology* 200, no. 4 (2009): 357–364.

15. Pearlstein et al., "Postpartum depression," 357–364.

16. Aleeca F. Bell, and Ewa Andersson, "The birth experience and women's postnatal depression: A systematic review," *Midwifery* 39 (2016): 112–123.

17. Center for Disease Control and Prevention, "Identifying Maternal Depression. Accessed November 21, 2020. https://www.cdc.gov/reproductivehealth/vital-signs/identifying-maternal-depression/index.html.

18. Michel Foucault, *Discipline and Punish: The Birth of the Prison.* Vintage, 2012.

19. Ian M. Paul, Danielle S. Downs, Eric W. Schaefer, Jessica S. Beiler, and Carol S. Weisman, "Postpartum anxiety and maternal-infant health outcomes," *Pediatrics* 131, no. 4 (2013): e1218–e1224.

20. Debra K. Creedy, Ian M. Shochet, and Jan Horsfall, "Childbirth and the development of acute trauma symptoms: incidence and contributing factors," *Birth* 27, no. 2 (2000): 104–111.

21. Shashi Rai, Abhishek Pathak, and Indira Sharma, "Postpartum psychiatric disorders: Early diagnosis and management," *Indian Journal of Psychiatry* 57, no. Suppl 2 (2015): S216.

22. Jane Eliot Sewell, *Cesarean Section – A Brief History* (Bethesda, MD: National Library of Medicine, 1993). https://www.nlm.nih.gov/exhibition/cesarean/index.html.

23. Sewell, *Cesarean Section*; Jacqueline Wolf, *Cesarean Section: An American History of Risk, Technology, and Consequence* (Baltimore, MD: Johns Hopkins University Press, 2018).

24. Wolf, *Cesarean Section*; Sewell, *Cesarean Section*.

25. Sewell, *Cesarean Section*.

26. Amy Chasteen Miller and Thomas E. Shriver, "Women's childbirth preferences and practices in the United States," *Social Science & Medicine* 75, no. 4 (2012): 709–716; Natasha Preskey, "Why are women still refusing painkillers during childbirth? *Vice*. January 3, 2019. Accessed November 21, 2020. https://www.vice.com/en_us/article/439mvm/this-is-why-the-natural-birth-movement-isnt-slowing-down.

27. Jacqueline Howard, "C-section deliveries nearly doubled worldwide since 2000, study finds," *CNN*. October 11, 2018. https://www.cnn.com/2018/10/11/health/c-section-rates-study-parenting-without-borders-intl/index.html; Sewell, *Cesarean Section*.

28. O'Cathain Alicia, Thomas Kate, Walters Stephen, Nicholl Jon, and Kirkham Mavis, "Women's perceptions of informed choice in maternity care," *Midwifery* 18, no. 2. (2002): 136–144.

29. Sewell, *Cesarean Section*.

30. Louise Marie Roth and Megan M. Henley, "Unequal motherhood: Racial-ethnic and socioeconomic disparities in cesarean sections in the United States," *Social Problems* 59, no. 2 (2012): 207–227.

31. Kamila Mistry, Kathryn Fingar, and Anne Elixhauser, "Variation in the rate of cesarean section across U.S. Hospitals, 2013," *Healthcare Cost and Utilization Project*. 2016. https://www.hcup-us.ahrq.gov/reports/statbrief.s/sb211-Hospital-Variation-C-sections-2013.pdf.

32. Adam Starkley, "Kate Hudson hit with backlash after saying having a c-section was 'lazy'," Metro. September 14, 2017. https://metro.co.uk/2017/09/14/kate-hudson-hit-with-backlash-after-saying-having-a-c-section-was-lazy-6928815/.

33. N.A., "Celebrity C-sections: Guess who's too posh to push," *Orlando Sentinel*. N.d. Accessed November 20, 2020. https://www.orlandosentinel.com/features/family/orl-celebrities-csections-moms-photos-photogallery.html.

34. Mark Reynolds, "Why Kate lied about Mia's birth," *Daily Mail*. N.d. Accessed November 20, 2020. https://www.dailymail.co.uk/tvshowbiz/article-300032/Why-Kate-lied-Mias-birth.html.

35. World Health Organization, "Monitoring emergency obstetric care," Accessed February 5, 2021. https://apps.who.int/iris/bitstream/handle/10665/44121/9789241547734_eng.pdf;jsessionid=19D4C0CF81B953E872746DF9A32FD7E4?sequence=1; George Molina, Thomas G. Weiser, Stuart R. Lipsitz, Micaela M. Esquivel, Tarsicio Uribe-Leitz, Tej Azad, Neel Shah et al., "Relationship between cesarean delivery rate and maternal and neonatal mortality," *Jama* 314, no. 21 (2015): 2263–2270.

36. Bonnie Fox and Diana Worts, "Revisiting the critique of medicalized childbirth: A contribution to the sociology of birth," *Gender & Society* 13, no. 3 (1999): 326–346; James McIntosh, "Models of childbirth and social class: A study of 80 working-class primigravidae," In *Midwives, Research and Childbirth*, 189–214 (Boston, MA: Springer, 1989; Margaret K. Nelson, "Working-class women, middle-class women, and models of childbirth," *Social Problems* 30, no. 3 (1983): 284–297.

Chapter 6

"I Just Hated Him"

The Impact of Trauma on Women's Relationships

Meghan's water broke at thirty-seven weeks when she was getting up from the couch. She did not experience any contractions. When she arrived at the hospital, her cervix was "not dilated at all." The doctor gave her medication, the name of which she cannot recall, to start contractions. After twelve hours, she had progressed to six centimeters, so the staff suggested that she have Pitocin and an epidural. Meghan has scoliosis so the anesthesiologist had a difficult time administering the analgesia. As a result, Meghan was only numb on one side of her body. After she screamed in pain, the staff brought in the lead anesthesiologist who was able to administer the epidural properly.

Over the next few hours, Meghan's cervix dilated to ten centimeters and she began to push. For four hours, she struggled in this manner but made little progress. Her body started to wear down. She was "so tired" that she was "falling asleep between my contractions." The team decided to prepare Meghan for a cesarean. As briefly discussed in chapter 1, Meghan had difficulty both in the staff's failing to consider her latex allergy and listening to her pleas to fix a poorly administered epidural.

Finally, she was brought to a recovery room. Nearly five hours later, she was able to see her baby. Unfortunately, Sandra was also struggling. Her lungs were not fully developed. She had a heart condition that required emergency surgery seventeen hours after birth. Then, after they were both finally discharged from the hospital, Meghan had to return to the emergency room, because she was severely anemic and proved to be bleeding internally.

While all of these experiences are objectively traumatic, Meghan remains plagued by the way she was treated by her medical team. A nurse threatened that they would take her baby from her if she "didn't figure out how to fucking breastfeed" and she was "manhandled by the lactation consultant" who just "grabbed my boob and started doing hand compressions . . . She didn't ask."

As a result of her physical trauma and the emotional struggles she had following her cesarean, Meghan had a difficult time caring for her baby, "Sometimes I don't think she's mine." Her husband, Justin, stepped in. He and Sandra bonded tightly during this time which led Meghan to "not like him very much because all I wanted was the baby to like me more than him." In retrospect, Meghan has "mad respect for Justin" because of the way he took care of them both, but at the time she "hated him . . . I hated him because it was so easy for him to like her."

In chapter 5, I explored the psychological impact of traumatic birth and the cultural forces that exacerbate these struggles. In this chapter, I examine how traumatic childbirth impacts women's relationships to their babies and families and how ideological and structural barriers to accessing postpartum care worsen these challenges.

As we have covered thus far in this book, institutions use time, space, and routine to discipline those within their reach.[1] In the case of mothers with difficult childbirth, these processes can be particularly injurious. The limitations of time can lead to poor interactions with staff that exacerbate trauma. The spatial structure that separates women from their babies in the NICU causes further harm. The taken-for-granted routines of care can restrict women's access to needed support. The operation of these processes reflects a deeply seated system of knowledge. This knowledge not only shapes time, space, and routine; it establishes what is normal and right for participants within the institution. Doctors, nurses, and even mothers are affected by these ideologies.

As a result of experiencing a difficult childbirth and the surmounting injury of institutional control, mothers struggle. They experience profound mental health challenges following childbirth. In the previous chapter, we examined how the internalization of knowledge about ideal childbirth causes psychological harm for women and separates them from other mothers. Here we further investigate the mental injury to mothers through consideration of postnatal care and the impact of trauma on mothers' relationships to their children and partners.

A GENEALOGY OF POSTNATAL CARE IN THE UNITED STATES

In chapter 2, I presented a brief genealogy of obstetric medicine in the United States. Here I offer the same look at postpartum care for mothers. As with obstetrics in general, postnatal support for mothers has varied significantly based on the dominant ideologies (or knowledges) of the time.

Prior to the nineteenth century, births primarily took place in the home. So too did the care of mothers after childbirth. For those who could afford it, families often hired caregivers to attend to new mothers. Others relied on the women in their social circles to support them.[2] As childbirth moved to hospitals and from midwifery to obstetric care in the 1900s, postpartum care also became medicalized. According to nurse and PhD researcher Louise K. Martell, nurses, the primary agents of postpartum care at this time, "rigidly controlled women's postpartum experiences and treated women as if they were ill."[3] Women resided in the hospital for approximately two weeks. During this time, babies were roomed apart from their mothers in hospital nurseries and only visited for planned nursing sessions. Women were expected to be docile and acquiesce to "hospital routine without question."[4]

During World War II, the length of hospital-based postpartum care decreased as hospitals faced staffing shortages as a result of the conflict. Birth wards were often overcrowded and, as such, some physicians sought to shorten postnatal care to three to five days while others questioned if such a change was safe for mothers.[5] These doctors feared fragile, white middle-class women would experience uterine prolapse or other poor outcomes if they were mobile so quickly following childbirth. As mentioned in chapter 2, social convention at the time contended that financially secure white women were more fragile than working-class white women or women of color. One physician in New Orleans used the success of Black women in postnatal mobility as evidence that such movement was safe and conducted an "early ambulation" study on white women concluding that postnatal mobility was safe.[6] This further challenged the broader treatment of women in the postnatal period as unwell.

The 1940s, then, brought initial consideration of the continued practice of separating mothers from their newborns. Neonatologists questioned whether early connection to mothers could improve child wellness and development and, accordingly, experimented with the practice of having infants "room-in" with their mothers.[7] In this model, mothers kept their infants by their bedside and served as their primary caretakers. Though rooming-in had its roots in this period, it remained a unique and uncommon practice.[8]

As with the broader medicalization of childbirth, the natural birth movement pushed back against standard practices in postnatal care. Adherents challenged the ways that wealthy white women were treated better than women of color and pushed back against the tradition of separating women from their infants and families.[9] These efforts, combined with scholarship that suggested child development is dependent on early bonding with mothers ultimately led to a model of postnatal care that included the entire family.[10] By the 1980s, fathers and siblings were permitted to be with mothers following birth. The standard practice shifted to allow infants and mothers (without extenuating healthcare needs) to room-in together. This shift also further reduced the time women stayed in the hospital following birth. Most women went home within two days of giving birth and received in-home or clinic-based follow-up care by nurses.[11] Such changes also saved hospitals money and freed up the demands on staff, further entrenching this change.

Today some scholars suggest that continued reduction of postpartum care has become a situation of "neglect." Such scholars as nurse and PhD research team Ching-Yu Cheng, Eileen Fowles, and Lorraine Walker contend that current efforts at postnatal care fail to provide adequate support to new mothers. They argue that the current practice of sending women home shortly after birth and then limiting additional care to a single six-week visit is insufficient, especially considering that this visit is restricted to examining a woman's physical healing and providing information about contraceptives. As we will discuss throughout in this chapter, women—especially those who experienced birth trauma—agree that this postpartum visit is insufficient to meet their needs for information about mental health, physical, and childcare.[12]

IMPACT OF TRAUMATIC BIRTH EXPERIENCES ON MOTHERS' RELATIONSHIPS WITH THEIR INFANTS

As introduced in the previous chapter, mental health challenges following childbirth are typically considered based on their type and severity. In his review article, Ian Brockington categorizes these challenges as postpartum depression, posttraumatic stress disorder, anxiety disorders, and "obsession of child harm."[13] Regardless of type, parental mental health challenges often impact parents' ability to care for their infants. While different ailments impact this relationship in distinct ways, infants are at risk when parents are mentally unwell and unable to access care. This section will examine different mental health challenges experienced by the women we talked with and their impact on the parent-child relationship. It is worth noting that I am not attempting to diagnose the women in my sample. Rather, I seek to showcase the impact the symptoms associated with each mental health struggle have on women's relationships to their infants.

Postpartum Depression

Postpartum depression (PPD) can influence the nature of the maternal-infant relationship and impact infant development. Women who suffer from PPD report greater challenges with responding to their child's needs or they may engage aggressively or even with hostility toward their children.[14] Postpartum depression affects approximately 15 percent of mothers.[15] This number is likely a severe underestimate due to both mothers' under-reporting and doctors' under- or misdiagnosis.[16]

As was mentioned at the start of this chapter, Meghan recalls feeling disconnected from her infant once they were able to return home from their hospital stays, which she attributes to postpartum depression. Reflecting on the early days with Sandra at home, Meghan remembers, "I had no idea, like, why this creature was in my life and why it wouldn't go away . . . I wanted, like, literally nothing to do with her for the first three weeks after she was born."

Like Meghan, Renee also believes she struggled with PPD but was not officially diagnosed as such. Renee feels a disconnect from her daughter, "I feel like I didn't give birth to her and I feel like she's a friend who I picked up from the bus station." Also, like Meghan, Renee wrestles with feelings of antagonism toward her daughter, whom she loves dearly. She remembers,

> It came to a head . . . I think it was like two weeks postpartum . . . I don't know what triggered it but there's a whole period of time I just don't remember. I just don't fucking remember. But I remember sitting on the bed and I remember I told Diane [her wife] that I wanted somebody to care about me and I wanted somebody to care about me more than Susan [her daughter] and, um, I just started screaming . . . And I just fucking lost my ever-loving shit. I started throwing furniture. I started screaming . . . I took Susan's bassinet, and I threw it across the room and I just completely destroyed our bedroom . . . There was never one point in time where I wanted to kill Susan. But I didn't want her to be around anymore and if that meant that she had died, I think at that point. I, ok, if that would, if that's what would make her not be around me anymore . . .

Responses to infants, such as Meghan's, Renee's, and other women who struggle with these aspects of PPD, can negatively impact the child's intellectual and social development as they rely on parental cues for the progression of these skills. Infants whose mothers have PPD experience higher rates of cognitive delays, insecure attachment, are more likely to struggle with anxiety, hyperactivity, or other behavioral problems as they age.[17] While many may blame the sufferers and survivors of postpartum mental health challenges for their behavior, the truth is that it is the lack of structural and cultural support that exacerbates these problems.

Postpartum Anxiety

Like PPD, postpartum anxiety (PPA) can cause severe distress for mothers and impact their relationship with their infant. Often considered to be a symptom of PPD, PPA has received less research attention. Women who

experience postpartum anxiety often struggle with persistent, severe feelings
of worry or dread. They often have difficulty sleeping or reduced appetite.[18]

As with postpartum depression, few women in our sample were diagnosed
with or sought treatment for postpartum anxiety. Yet, in their stories, they
shared many struggles associated with the symptoms of this impairment. For
example, Lisa feared her child had been damaged by not being held immediately following birth. For Lisa, this fear is specifically tied to the belief that
he may develop autism because of this experience. She says, "I have this
huge fear that my baby's going to be autistic and, so now every time that he
like doesn't make eye contact with me then I have this huge fear and I work
myself up into this big ball of anxiety . . . I'm sure there are a million things
to worry about when you're just a regular mom, but now there's like another
layer of things, you know?" Lisa's statement is particularly powerful. She
is anxious about her son's wellbeing fearing that the difficult childbirth will
have future impacts on his health. And she concurrently expresses that she is
not a "regular mom." Lisa is concurrently plagued with significant feelings of
guilt about her body's perceived "failure" to nurture him.

Sometimes postpartum anxiety can also manifest as obsessive-compulsive
disorder (OCD). When experiencing OCD, mothers often struggle with
intrusive thoughts, often of bad things happening to their babies or even of
them causing said harm. They may try to mitigate the associated anxiety with
compulsions, such as obsessive cleaning, checking on their infant or objects
around the home, cleaning, hoarding, and other rituals. Mothers who struggle
with postnatal OCD often fear being alone with their child.

Posttraumatic Stress Disorder

Posttraumatic stress disorder often manifests in mothers being withdrawn,
unable to connect with their child or, for some women, anger and hyper-
arousal.[19] PTSD is also often concurrent with postpartum depression, so many
women may also experience the symptoms outlined above.[20]

As with other mental health struggles following childbirth, postnatal
PTSD is associated with negative connection to infants. For example, at six
months postpartum, higher postnatal PTSD symptom scores in mothers were
associated with lower quality interactions with their infants.[21] The percentage
of mothers who were sensitive to their child's needs and had a cooperative
infant is also significantly lower among women experiencing symptoms of
posttraumatic stress.[22] Similar results were reported by Nancy Feeley, professor of nursing at McGill University, and her research team, who found that
mothers of preterm infants with higher postpartum PTSD symptoms were
less sensitive and effective at structuring interactions with their infant at six
months postpartum.[23] Furthermore, psychology professors Chiara Ionio and

Paola Di Blasio reported that postpartum PTSD symptoms were associated with mothers not looking directly at their infant, intruding in child's independent play, and describing their infant in a negative way at three months postpartum.[24]

One woman in our sample, Summer, struggled with feeling both disconnected from and hostile toward her son. Summer's labor lasted over forty-eight hours. During this time, her son's "heart rate was becoming an issue and his oxygen level." Yet, Summer was able to deliver vaginally. For Summer, one of the most difficult parts of her birth and early parenthood was nursing. She developed mastitis within the first week of his delivery. Mastitis occurs when breast tissue becomes inflamed and, often, infected. The condition can be incredibly painful and also cause the mother to experience flu-like symptoms: fever and chills.[25] In Summer's case, the infection was so extreme that she had to stop breastfeeding "or else run the risk of losing a breast because my mastitis was so severe." She was put on antibiotics but still recalls the extensive pain she felt, "I remember laying in the bathtub just crying because of how owie it was." After her son's birth, she struggled with undiagnosed postpartum mental health challenges. She recalls,

> I couldn't make eye contact with my son. I felt guilty that I could not make eye contact with him . . . And, like, sometimes I feel like he would want me to look at him and I can still remember these times, even though he is going on ten, it's crazy . . . Where I feel like he would want me to look at him, but I just couldn't and then he would cry because he wanted me to look at him. Or something like that. Or, he would be crying, and he wanted me to look at him and I couldn't do that.

Like many people who struggle with postnatal trauma, Summer felt distant from and antagonistic toward her son following his birth.

Kathy delivered her baby after a long labor and a transfer from an attempted home birth to the hospital. She also had a difficult time with nursing and was unable to find adequate support. Like Summer, Kathy experienced feelings of aggression toward her child following her traumatic birth. She shared, "I had this really strong urge to throw him. I wanted to make him go away." In this particular event, Kathy woke her husband and told him, "You have to take him. I'm afraid of what I might do."

Postnatal PTSD has been associated with troubling mother-infant relationships and, possibly due to said relationships, child temperament later in childhood. For example, in their longitudinal study, Garthus-Niegel, Ayers, Martini, von Soest, and Eberhard-Gran found that postnatal PTSD was connected with poor social-emotional development for children at two years and that this was especially pronounced for boys and infants who had challenging temperaments.[26] Maternal postnatal PTSD is also correlated with cognitive development in toddlerhood.[27]

IMPACT ON MOTHERS' RELATIONSHIPS
WITH OTHER CHILDREN

The experience of trauma during childbirth and associated mental health challenges does not only impact a mother's relationship to the child born during the traumatic birth. Rather, it also affects the relationship she has to her other children both during the experience and in more lasting ways. Existing research indicates that many women who experienced traumatic births feel particularly protective of their infants, sometimes to the detriment of their other children.[28] This was true of the women we interviewed who discussed the impact of their difficult or traumatic childbirth on their older children; they felt that they prioritized the child born during the difficult birth in ways that caused damage to their relationships to older children.

When Dee was thirty-two-weeks pregnant, she developed preeclampsia and associated liver problems. As a result, she delivered her son prematurely after being flown via air ambulance to a nearby urban hospital. Dee believes that her traumatic birth experience "really hurt Jack and I's relationship." Before her new baby was born, she had been a stay-at-home mom with their eldest. "For three years I was home with him . . . I took care of all his needs. I gave him attention and all that sort of stuff." Then, suddenly, Jack was met with a new baby and a mom who needed to heal from trauma. Dee recalls, "Not only is there this other baby but I'm dealing with this sense of failure, the postpartum depression." She recalls that Jack lashed out—he was "jealous," and his behavior further caused Dee to "question my abilities as a mother . . . because he wouldn't listen to me." Dee believes that "he was acting out because he was jealous and because he was three" but this new dynamic really impacted their relationship. Dee recalls, "it changed my relationship with him so much because I kind of was apathetic at that time like about so many things. I could not even make myself make the effort to follow through, I would just be like 'I guess he's not going to do that and there's nothing I can do about it' . . . I feel like I let him down, I feel like it hurt his and mine relationship."

Joan delivered her baby early following a loss of amniotic fluid. Like Dee, she found herself "very protective" of her newborn. He was born early after experiencing distress when her amniotic fluid began to leak. The anxiety surrounding his birth led Joan to make a "little bubble" of the two of them and keep her older kids "away" so that they would not "bother or hurt" their young sibling.

There is not much research on the impact of traumatic childbirth on women's relationships to existing children. However, given the heightened experiences of anxiety about infants born from traumatic births, it seems likely these experiences are common. The research that has been done focuses on the impact of postnatal trauma on future children. It finds that women who have a traumatic birth fear future pregnancy and childbirth.[29] When they do have subsequent kids, women report being more anxious and protective of those born during traumatic circumstances.[30]

IMPACT ON RELATIONSHIP WITH PARTNER

The women we interviewed also talked at length of the impact their traumatic delivery had on their relationships to their partners. The two most common responses were a lack of interest in sex and feelings of resentment toward their partners.

Most of the women we talked to expressed difficulty with sex following their traumatic birth. Existing research suggests that these feelings are quite common and may be caused by women's fear of becoming pregnant, being reminded of the event, having flashbacks during sexual engagement, or simply not wanting to be touched.[31]

The women we interviewed reported feeling a lack of desire or, for some, fear. Lisa, for example, felt like her relationship to her husband became more like that of a "patient," even when she returned home from the hospital. She says that she has "such fear about becoming pregnant" that she does not want to have sex with her husband, "there's like no intimacy because I'm afraid." She explains that this fear is exacerbate because she is "sad all the time and irritable." A small part of her is fearful that she will "be like a statistic of couples who have a premature infant or a sick baby . . . and get divorced." Samantha, too, recalls trying to avoid sexual intimacy with her husband. She said, "It just makes me uncomfortable. I have flashbacks to my time in the hospital when he touches me. I feel too vulnerable, maybe even fragile. It doesn't make for a great experience."

Beyond affecting their sex life, women expressed that their traumatic birth caused problems with resentment in their relationship to their partners. Meghan says that even at the time of our interview, years after her daughter's birth, she and her husband "fight about the fact that Sandra likes him more than me." Meghan feels resentful of her husband and daughter's relationship. Her husband responds to her challenge by saying she is "being self-deprecating and I need to be quiet." She recalls that in the early days following her daughter's delivery, she "hated him." She remembers, "he just saw this tiny little creature and was like 'I love you, you're my favorite person in the whole world.'" Meghan resented him because "this isn't how it's supposed to work. I'm supposed to have the instantaneous bond. Not you, you asshole."

Renee also resented her wife, but largely because she felt that Susan dismissed the intensity of Renee's postpartum struggles. Renee felt like the people in her life "were just trying to diminish what was going on" with her emotional health. She felt as though Susan was also "on the side of the minimizer." Though Renee recognizes that Susan was responding this way "out of love" instead, Renee "really resented her for that."

Meghan and Renee are not alone. Existing research also suggests that traumatic childbirth impacts women's relationships with their partners and their sex drive.[32] For example, researchers Karen Nicolls and Susan Ayers interviewed couples following traumatic births. They found that the women in their sample reported feeling deserted by their partners when they returned to work. Their participants also discussed a need to avoid sexual intercourse because it reminded them of their birth trauma, potentially leading to flashbacks, because they felt they had to protect their "battered and bashed" bodies, and due to a fear of pregnancy.[33] In a second interview project led by psychologist Susan Ayers, researchers found that women reported their relationships suffered as a result of several factors: women's decreased self-esteem, women's loss of interest in sex, arguments about the birth experience, women's sense of blame toward their partners for events during the birth, and women spending less time with their partners. None of their participants reported that their birth trauma positively impacted their relationship with their partners.[34]

ACCESS TO POSTPARTUM MENTAL HEALTH CARE

Despite the severity of postpartum mental health disorders, new mothers are underserved. Psychiatric disorders among new mothers are underreported and undertreated and women lack access to care.[35]

Currently, in the United States, postpartum care typically takes the form of a visit to the obstetrician six weeks after delivery.[36] The focus of this appointment is to verify that the mother is physically healing well and to discuss contraceptives.[37] While some doctors will ask women about their mental health, this is not the primary concern of the appointment. Women often feel dissatisfied with postnatal care.[38]

For example, Dr. Carolyn R. Kline, MD, MPH and her research team conducted focus groups with new mothers in the first fifteen months postpartum. They also held focus groups with midwives and doctors who focused on obstetric and gynecological care. In their sample, approximately 30 percent of women reported that they did not feel like their concerns are met at their six-week postnatal doctors' visits and that they felt largely unprepared for early motherhood.[39] Specifically, women report wanting to discuss social issues such as balancing their new role as mother with their existing roles. They desired to talk about how to care for their newborn baby and get tips on breastfeeding. Mothers sought to discuss sex, including topics such as change in level of desire or physical changes resulting from childbirth. Mothers also hoped that this postnatal visit would offer an opportunity to find emotional and mental support for things like depression, self-care, feelings about their changing bodies, and other such experiences.

The women we interviewed also felt that their needs were not met at the six-week follow-up appointment. Samantha, for example, reflects on these themes with regard to her doctor's visit. She says, "Care for mothers after their babies are born needs to be better. I saw my doctor once and barely even knew what to think or ask, I was so tired." Later in the interview, Samantha returns to this topic, "Care for mothers after birth needs to include emotional support." Like the women in Kline et al.'s study, Samantha pointed to the care she really needed from her doctor at this time. She went to her appointment thinking it would be a space to "talk" and "process" but failed to get the assistance she needed.

Dee also felt that postpartum care should include a conversation with women about their mental health. Pointing to the effects of mental health on relationships, Dee questions why doctors are not "checking on the parent's relationships and . . . the relationships with the kids. You know what I mean?"

The women we interviewed further felt abandoned by their care team after delivering their children. One of our interviewees, Sue, explains this sentiment saying,

> I felt very little concern from the practice here in Springfield that I had left. I had this baby, and they were like, "ok, we're done" . . . I never saw the doctors again . . . It felt like a very jarring transition . . . I guess at the end of the day I never felt like I had a doctor who was checking in with me. I had people who were for the baby, or like the delivery piece, but no one for the, whole arc of it, for the mom. And that is not ideal. But I don't know what the solution is.

Kathy had similar feelings regarding the postpartum care she received from her obstetrician. She recalls, "I had two postpartum visits and then she was gone." Kathy felt discarded and unsupported.

While the above examples are not clearly focused just on postnatal mental health care, issues such as postpartum depression, anxiety, and postnatal post-traumatic stress disorder need to be part of the aftercare treatment for new mothers. Yet, despite the prevalence of these struggles, women are largely dismissed by their doctors following the delivery of their babies. The lack of mental health care is, in part, a reflection of cultural norms and expectations. Doctors and mothers often see depression and anxiety as a so-called "normal" part of the postpartum period—a typical response to hormonal, physical, and environmental changes. We see this in Kathy when she says her anxiety "could just be a mom thing." The normalization of mental health struggles postpartum also occurs among healthcare professionals who often see it as a typical consequence of childbirth.[40]

Because postpartum care is difficult to access, mothers have to take the initiative to do so themselves. This is something that someone struggling with postpartum depression, anxiety, or trauma may be unable to do. Beyond this structural barrier, postnatal health care is often not covered by insurance, making it only available to wealthy mothers. Even for people who can afford mental health care, there are stigmas and fears associated with treatment that may prevent one from seeking help. Mothers may be embarrassed they need assistance or they may worry it will alert child protective services that something is wrong.

Even when people are able to find the time, money, and mental capacity to seek help, they often face yet another barrier: a lack of available mental health professionals in rural communities. While rates of postpartum mental health care for women in the United States are low in general, they are even more restricted for women in rural communities.[41] As with most medical professionals, psychologists and therapists tend to be concentrated in urban or suburban areas.[42] This rural mental healthcare shortage results in part from the isolation care providers face: They are tasked with providing care for people without support staff such as case managers or even colleagues to turn to for help.[43]

In chapter 3, I discussed Joan's experience in seeking to access postpartum care. In response to persistent mental health struggles, she called her doctor who referred her to several therapists but found that "there's a six-month wait list to get in." But Joan was suffering; six months was too long to wait, "That was a struggle I had in this area, was just getting in to see someone." Renee, too, was unable to access adequate mental health support following her daughter's birth. At the time of our interview, her daughter was four months old and, though Renee faced exorbitant challenges from what she believed to be postpartum depression, she still had not been able to obtain psychological care.

Many psychologists opt not to practice in rural areas because they rely on insurance for their client's services, and a disproportionate number of women in rural communities are on Medicaid or go without insurance. Furthermore, federal policy only guarantees Medicaid for sixty days following childbirth and, depending on their state's policy, women on Medicaid may lose coverage after two months postpartum.[44]

It is worth mentioning that mothers' mental health is also undermined by abysmal family leave policies. In the United States, parental leave is covered under the Family and Medical Leave (FMLA) program which gives employees up to twelve weeks of unpaid leave. During this time, their jobs and benefits are protected.[45] While employers may provide some paid leave options or extended time, these expanded leave programs are predominately only available to people in high-income earning jobs.

Many new mothers are not even eligible for FMLA. In order to qualify, one needs to have worked at their current place of employment for more than 1,760 hours at their job in the year prior. Thus, people in new jobs are ineligible. FMLA is also only applicable for people who work at businesses with over fifty employees, eliminating people who work in small companies from eligibility. Those fifty employees also need to live within 75 miles of the office, excluding people who work at all or mostly remote businesses.[46]

For context, the Organization of Economic Cooperation and Development compared forty-one wealthy nations and found that the United States ranks last in terms of paid leave for new parents. While the United States does not guarantee any paid leave, the top-ranked nation, Estonia, offers eighty-six weeks of paid leave for new parents. Nine countries (Austria, Bulgaria, Hungary, Japan, Latvia, Lithuania, Norway, Slovakia, and Slovenia) offer over a year of paid leave.[47] Some nations also permit leave to begin in the last weeks of pregnancy. In Norway, for example, women are given three weeks of leave prior to their due date.[48]

As a result of the United States' dreadful leave policies, women lack the time to heal both physically and mentally from childbirth. They are unable to adapt to their changing bodies and altered lives. Particularly injured are low-income mothers who often have to return to work immediately following or soon after their child's birth simply to survive.[49]

CONCLUSION

Traumatic childbirth and associated mental health challenges have significant impacts on women's relationships. Of the women we talked to, the most common effects were on their relationship to their child, their partners, and their existing children. While some women feared they would harm their children, most experienced increased anxiety around their child's safety. This rippled into their relationships with existing children. The women we interviewed also felt resentment toward their partners and a loss of interest in sex.

In the previous chapters, I explored how both the structures and ideologies in place hurt women. Here, again, we find this same process of power perpetuating trauma. Women are unable to access postpartum mental health care. The structure of our healthcare system is such that there are simply not enough providers in rural areas. Therefore, those that do exist locally do not have time available to provide urgent care for new mothers. Again, Foucault's contention that time, space, and routine are all subtle ways institutions exert power over citizens resonates.

The mental anguish of women is real. It is not their fault. It is informed, fed, and bred by the ideological structures in society that tell women they are not enough, that they failed, that they are bad mothers. This is, again, evidence of the subtle methods through which power operates.

NOTES

1. Michel Foucault, *Discipline and Punish: The Birth of the Prison* (Vintage, 2012).

2. Louise Martell, "The hospital and the postpartum experience: A historical analysis," *Journal of Obstetric, Gynecologic, and Neonatal Nursing* 29, no. 1 (2000): 65–72.

3. Martell, "The hospital and postpartum experience," 65–72; Louise Martell, "Maternity care during the post–world war II baby boom," *Western Journal of Nursing Research* 21 (1999): 387–404.

4. Martell, "The hospital and postpartum experience," 65–72; Louise Martell, "Maternity care during the post–world war II baby boom," 387–404.

5. Martell, "The hospital and postpartum experience," 65–72.

6. Martell, "The hospital and postpartum experience," 65–72; Wm. Guerriero, "Early controlled ambulation in the Puerperium," *American Journal of Obstetrics and Gynecology* 51 (1948): 312–313.

7. Martell, "The hospital and postpartum experience," 65–72.

8. Martell, "The hospital and postpartum experience," 65–72.

9. Martell, "The hospital and postpartum experience," 65–72.

10. Martell, "The hospital and postpartum experience," 65–72; Marshall Klaus, Richard Jerauld, Nancy Kreger, Willie McAlphine, Meredith Steffa, and John Kennell, "Maternal attachment – Importance of first post-partum days," *The New England Journal of Medicine* 286 (1972): 460–463.

11. Martell, "The hospital and postpartum experience," 65–72.

12. Ching-Yu Cheng, Eileen R. Fowles, and Lorraine O. Walker, "Postpartum maternal health care in the United States: A critical review," *The Journal of Perinatal Education* 15, no. 3 (2006): 34.

13. Ian Brockington, "Diagnosis and management of post-partum disorders: A review," *World Psychiatry* 3, no. 2 (2004): 89.

14. Riikka Korja, Elina Savonlahti, Sari Ahlqvist-Björkroth, Suvi Stolt, Leena Haataja, Helena Lapinleimu, Jorma Piha, Liisa Lehtonen, and PIPARI Study Group, "Maternal depression is associated with mother-infant interaction in preterm infants," *Acta Paediatrica* 97, no. 6 (2008): 724–730; Cheryl Beck, "Postpartum depressed mothers' experiences interacting with their children," *Nursing Research*

45, no. 2 (1996): 98–104; Lynne Murray, Peter Cooper, and Alison Hipwell. "Mental health of parents caring for infants," *Archives of Women's Mental Health* 6, no. 2 (2003): s71–s77.

15. Teri Pearlstein, Margaret Howard, Amy Salisbury, and Caron Zlotnick, "Postpartum depression," *American Journal of Obstetrics and Gynecology* 200, no. 4 (2009): 357–364.

16. Grace Evins, James Theofrastous, and Shelley Galvin, "Postpartum depression: A comparison of screening and routine clinical evaluation," *American Journal of Obstetrics and Gynecology* 182, no. 5 (2000): 1080–1082.

17. S. R. Cogill, H. L. Caplan, Heather Alexandra, Kay Mordecai Robson, and R. Kumar, "Impact of maternal postnatal depression on cognitive development of young children," *British Medical Journal (Clin Res Ed)* 292, no. 6529 (1986): 1165–1167; Carla Martins and Elizabeth A. Gaffan, "Effects of early maternal depression on patterns of infant–mother attachment: A meta-analytic investigation," *Journal of Child Psychology and Psychiatry* 41, no. 6 (2000): 737–746; Marilyn Essex, Marjorie H. Klein, Eunsuk Cho, and Ned H. Kalin, "Maternal stress beginning in infancy may sensitize children to later stress exposure: effects on cortisol and behavior," *Biological Psychiatry* 52, no. 8 (2002): 776–784; Dana Sinclair and Lynne Murray, "Effects of postnatal depression on children's adjustment to school," *The British Journal of Psychiatry* 172, no. 1 (1998): 58–63; R. M. Wrate, A. C. Rooney, P. F. Thomas, and J. L. Cox, "Postnatal depression and child development: A three-year follow-up study," *The British Journal of Psychiatry* 146, no. 6 (1985): 622–627.

18. Texas Children's Hospital, "Recognizing signs of postpartum anxiety," Accessed November 20, 2020. https://women.texaschildrens.org/blog/recognizing-signs-postpartum-anxiety.

19. Susan Garthus-Niegel, Susan Ayers, Julia Martini, Tilmann von Soest, and Malin Eberhard-Gran, "The impact of postpartum post-traumatic stress disorder symptoms on child development: A population-based, 2-year follow-up study," *Psychological Medicine*, 47 (2017): 161–170.

20. Garthus-Niegel et al., "The impact of postpartum post-traumatic stress disorder symptoms," 161–170.

21. Carole Muller-Nix, Margarita Forcada-Guex, Blaise Pierrehumbert, Lyne Jaunin, Ayala Borghini, and François Ansermet, "Prematurity, maternal stress and mother–child interactions," *Early Human Development* 79, no. 2 (2004): 145–158.

22. Margarita Forcada-Guex, Ayala Borghini, Blaise Pierrehumbert, François Ansermet, and Carole Muller-Nix, "Prematurity, maternal posttraumatic stress and consequences on the mother–infant relationship," *Early Human Development* 87, no. 1 (2011): 21–26.

23. Nancy Feeley, Phyllis Zelkowitz, Carole Cormier, Lyne Charbonneau, Annie Lacroix, and Apostolos Papageorgiou, "Posttraumatic stress among mothers of very low birthweight infants at 6 months after discharge from the neonatal intensive care unit," *Applied Nursing Research* 24, no. 2 (2011): 114–117.

24. Chiara Ionio and Paola Di Blasio, "Post-traumatic stress symptoms after childbirth and early mother–child interactions: An exploratory study," *Journal of Reproductive and Infant Psychology* 32, no. 2 (2014): 163–181.

25. The Mayo Clinic, "Mastitis," Accessed November 5, 2020. https://www.may oclinic.org/diseases-conditions/mastitis/symptoms-causes/syc-20374829.

26. Garthus-Niegel et al., "The impact of postpartum post-traumatic stress disorder symptoms," 161–170.

27. Ylva Parfitt, Susan Ayers, Alison Pike, D. C. Jessop, and Elizabeth Ford, "A prospective study of the parent–baby bond in men and women 15 months after birth," *Journal of Reproductive and Infant Psychology* 32, no. 5 (2014): 441–456.

28. Karen Nicholls and Susan Ayers, "Childbirth-related post-traumatic stress disorder in couples: A qualitative study," *British Journal of Health Psychology* 12, no. 4 (2007): 491–509.

29. Susan Ayers, "Fear of childbirth, postnatal post-traumatic stress disorder and midwifery care," *Midwifery* 30, no. 2 (2014): 145–148.

30. Susan Ayers, Andrew Eagle, and Helen Waring, "The effects of childbirth-related post-traumatic stress disorder on women and their relationships: A qualitative study," *Psychology, Health & Medicine* 11, no. 4 (2006): 389–398.

31. Rakime Elmir, Virginia Schmied, Lesley Wilkes, and Debra Jackson, "Women's perceptions and experiences of a traumatic birth: A meta-ethnography." *Journal of Advanced Nursing* 66, no. 10 (2010): 2142–2153; Nicholls and Ayers, "Childbirth-related post-traumatic stress disorder," 491–509; Ayers et al., "The effects of postnatal PTSD," 389–398.

32. Ayers et al., "The effects of postnatal PTSD," 389–398.

33. Nicholls and Ayers, "Childbirth-related post-traumatic stress disorder," 491–509.

34. Ayers et al., "The effects of postnatal PTSD," 389–398.

35. Oriana Vesga-Lopez, Carlos Blanco, Katherine Keyes, Mark Olfson, Bridget F. Grant, and Deborah S. Hasin, "Psychiatric disorders in pregnant and postpartum women in the United States," *Archives of General Psychiatry* 65, no. 7 (2008): 805–815; Vesga-Lopez et al., "Psychiatric disorders in pregnant and postpartum women," 805–815.

36. Ching-Yu Cheng, Eileen R. Fowles, and Lorraine O. Walker, "Postpartum maternal health care in the United States: A critical review," *The Journal of Perinatal Education* 15, no. 3 (2006): 34.

37. Cheng et al., "Continuing education module," 34–42.

38. Eugene R. Declercq, Carol Sakala, Maureen P. Corry, S. Applebaum, and Peter Risher, "Listening to mothers: Report of the first national US survey of women's childbearing experiences," *New York* (2002).

39. Cheng et al., "Continuing education module," 34–42; Declercq et al., "Listening to mothers."

40. Vesga-Lopez et al., "Psychiatric disorders in pregnant and postpartum women," 805–815.

41. Center for Medicare and Medicaid Service, "Improving access to maternal health care in rural communities," 2019, Accessed November 5, 2020. https://ww w.cms.gov/About-CMS/Agency-Information/OMH/equity-initiatives/rural-health/ 09032019-Maternal-Health-Care-in-Rural-Communities.pdf.

42. David Levine, "How much of a struggle is it to get mental health care in rural areas?" *U.S. News and World Report,* 2018 April 20. Accessed November 5, 2020.

https://health.usnews.com/health-care/patient-advice/articles/2018-04-20/how-much
-of-a-struggle-is-it-to-get-mental-health-care-in-rural-areas.

43. David Levine, "How much of a struggle is it to get mental health care in rural areas?"

44. "Improving Access to Maternal Health Care in Rural Communities," Center for Medicare and Medicaid Service, "Maternal and Obstetric care challenges in rural America," National Advisory Committee on Rural Health and Human Services. Accessed November 5, 2020. https://www.hrsa.gov/sites/default/files/hrsa/advisory-committees/rural/publications/2020-maternal-obstetric-care-challenges.pdf.

45. "Family and Medical Leave (FMLA)," United States Department of Labor. Accessed November 5, 2020. https://www.dol.gov/general/topic/benefits-leave/fmla.

46. "Family and Medical Leave (FMLA)," United States Department of Labor.

47. Gretchen Livingston and Thomas, Deja. "Among 41 countries, only U.S. lacks paid parental leave," Pew Research Center. December 16, 2019. Accessed November 5th, 2020. https://www.pewresearch.org/fact-tank/2019/12/16/u-s-lacks-mandated-paid-parental-leave/.

48. Organization of Economic Cooperation and Development, "Parental Leave Systems," Accessed February 8, 2021. https://www.oecd.org/els/soc/PF2_1_Parental_leave_systems.pdf.

49. Megan Shepherd-Banigan and Janice F. Bell, "Paid leave benefits among a national sample of working mothers with infants in the United States," *Maternal and Child Health Journal* 18, no. 1 (2014): 286–295. doi:10.1007/s10995-013-1264-3.

Chapter 7

"He Was So Supportive"

Using Power and Restructuring Obstetric Care

At thirty-five-weeks pregnant, Nancy was diagnosed with gestational diabetes. To complicate matters, her blood pressure began to rise and though she was "never diagnosed as preeclamptic" the doctors put Nancy on "modified bed rest." They also planned to do an induction at thirty-eight weeks if Nancy's labor had not started on its own.

Thirty-eight weeks arrived, and Nancy was given Cervidil, a drug used to instigate the cervix to ripen and launch labor. The drug did not have its intended effect, so they administered Pitocin, which causes uterine contractions. She remained in the hospital a full week, but her labor did not commence. The medical team was at a loss and planned to artificially help Nancy's water break the next day. However, during the night, her baby started to show signs of fetal distress. The medical team decided they needed to move quickly and perform a cesarean.

Having spent a week with the nurses and doctors at the hospital, Nancy felt differently about this turn of events than other women we talked with. She recalls thinking "I felt safe and secure which was terrifying at the same time," though it was "not the route I had hoped to end up on."

Despite saying she felt safe before the surgery, Nancy relates that she was very nervous during it. She was "shaking so bad" that she feared she would "vibrate right off" the operating table. When she made a comment to this effect, the anesthesiologist took it upon himself to help her calm down. He let her "pick our music that we wanted to listen to" and he talked her "through most of what was going on." She remembers feeling so supported by him that she "loved him."

After her son was finally born, he struggled with respiratory distress. As a result, Nancy was unable to hold him, and he was taken to the nursery. She forced her husband to follow. Despite being separated from her son, Nancy says that she "was not worried . . . because I knew he was getting the best possible care."

Nancy and her son were discharged from the hospital after several days. She says it was not until about three weeks later that the full force of her experience hit her. Nancy cries in our interview recalling how she and her husband talked together to try to process their experiences. While she does not feel the sense of betrayal that many of the women we interviewed did, she does spend a lot of time wondering how things could have ended up differently. If they had broken her water instead of waiting so long, would his lungs have been better?

While most of the other interviews we conducted focused on the events of the labor and both the positive and negative interactions with staff, Nancy's differed in the connection that she had with her medical team. Perhaps because she had gotten to know them so well in advance of her birth, she felt confident with them and their ability to care for her and her son. That proved to mitigate some of her pain as a consequence of the emergency situations that later developed. When we talked with Nancy about her experience, she said that she felt like she was well-informed about the events that transpired before and as they happened. This helped her maintain a level of confidence in her care. Her doctor and the nurses explained interventions prior to applying them and detailed the reasons for the choice.

Like the other women we interviewed, Nancy experienced objectively difficult or traumatizing events during her pregnancy. She had an emergency cesarean following a week-long stay at the hospital. Her son had difficulty breathing at birth and she did not get to meet him for several hours. She also has some lingering challenges. She questions some of the events that occurred and wonders if they could have been avoided. However, unlike most of the women we interviewed, she is not haunted by negative interactions with hospital staff. In some ways, it appears, this may have helped preserve elements of her emotional health.

Through the first six chapters of this book, I focused on the factors that cause or exacerbate postnatal trauma for mothers and the impact these experiences have on their mental health and relationships. In this chapter, I explore the moments when doctors got it right—when they exploited the fissures within the power-knowledge system. I then offer alternative knowledge, from the women in my sample, to improve obstetric care through claiming time, changing space, and altering routines. Finally, I present additional insights offered by Finland and Germany—their obstetric and mental healthcare systems, respectively—into how it may be possible to restructure obstetric care in the United States in a way that helps and supports mothers.

RESISTING THE INSTITUTIONAL AND
IDEOLOGICAL FORCES OF POWER

For Foucault, power is the "medium of change," the production of knowledge.[1] It is not a possession to be had but a tool to use. One does not have to be atop a hierarchy to exercise power but anyone within a power-knowledge system can resist and contribute to its transformation. However, Foucault's theorizing of social change is limiting and best extended by the work of key feminist philosophers. One, Susan Bordo deepens Foucault's analysis contending that, even though power is not possessed by any individual, it does not impact all people the same.[2] Rather, systems of power impact people in a variety of constellations based on factors, such as their race, gender, economic class, or age, to name a few. Bordo further emphasizes that resistance to existing power systems is constantly exerted by those "below" and that, in return, institutions and knowledge systems are "continually being penetrated and reconstructed by values, styles, and knowledges that have been developing and gathering strength, energy, and distinctiveness 'at the margins.'" She further argues that the associated change is slow, localized, and often small.[3]

Still, however, we lack a clear conception of *how* social change happens. In her recent work, Sara Ahmed offers insight into the way that "saying 'no'" to existing power structures serves concurrently to make visible its insidious operation, to warn women who will encounter them in the future, but also to push back against their operation—"the reproduction of what is being refused" in the ways that "no" causes "leaks" and can become "catchy" and "cause more trouble along the way." Ahmed contends that a "no" can serve to amplify the "nos" of others and build resistance.[4]

Taken together, Foucault, Bordo, and Ahmed could lead one to contend that by saying "no" to the existing power/knowledge system—by taking control over time, space, and routine—women and medical practitioners reconstruct power-knowledge systems or, at the very least, use power to make them visible and cause "leaks." In looking at the experiences of women in our sample, we find this to be the case. When practitioners *took time*, women felt heard, seen, and valued. When doctors made exceptions and *repatterned space* (such as allowing women to stay with their infants against protocol), they reduced mothers' pain. When they *rejected routine* and, instead, accounted for the specific needs of a given situation, they alleviated and prevented suffering.

In this chapter, then, I look at examples of successful interactions between practitioners and mothers. These moments were positive not in the ways that they reinforced and produced social knowledge but, in the opposite, in the ways that they resisted and pushed back against these systems, creating new knowledge and norms. I also present suggestions by mothers to improve care

and provide two examples of an alternative model for care, maternity care in
Finland and mental health care in Germany.

"I LOVE THIS MAN": TRAUMA MITIGATION
THROUGH TAKING TIME

Through all of the stories told by women for this project, one thing is clear:
direct, mindful, compassionate communication is key to leaving women
feeling positive about their birth experiences, even if they experienced an
extraordinarily challenging or scary process. In particular, women celebrated
when medical staff took the time to listen and answer their questions, treated
them like intellectual peers, recognized the emotions they were experiencing,
and generally treated them with kindness.

One doctor was celebrated by many women in our sample for the way he
took the time to explain processes to them and treated them as intelligent,
agentic, capable beings. Dr. Fischer is a young doctor, local to the community, with a large family of his own. He recalls that, during medical school,
he was told most doctors only listen to patients for eleven seconds before they
interrupt.[5] To this routine, he said "no" and committed to actively listen to his
clients. And, as is demonstrated by the women in our sample, this practice is
effective.

For example, Meghan recalls how Dr. Fischer dedicated time to listening to
her and clarifying her experiences during her second child's birth,

> Dr. Fischer was wonderful. He explained to me everything that was happening.
> He was very "This is what we're going to do" and he knew that I had gone
> through everything with Sandra and so he was very calming and reassuring . . .
> [He] kept asking, "Was I processing this okay? Was I getting through? Did I feel
> comfortable with what was happening?" And I was like "I don't feel comfort-
> able with the fact that he is coming early, but I feel comfortable with the fact
> that you guys know what you're doing and you're not pushing me into doing
> something that I don't want to do."

Throughout our interviews, women stressed how important it was to them
to know what was happening with their labors, their children, and their bodies. By taking the time to explain concerns, procedures, and to answer questions, Dr. Fischer mitigated the effects of frightening, powerless processes.

Women also celebrated Dr. Fischer because he treated them as intellectual peers. The mothers we interviewed report he often shared academic
articles with them or explained difficult procedures in intellectual, and not

condescending, ways. Kayla—who had two traumatic birth experiences—recalls how Dr. Fischer supported her through the days leading up to her delivery of her premature daughter,

> When he took over the care, he was so supportive, so knowledgeable . . . He was talking to us like partners . . . It was not, "Here's what we are going to do to you and your body." No, he was like, "Here is the situation. Here are the options. This is what I think should be happening, right?" . . . What he did, which is so cool of him, is, he's, "Well I know you're an academic and you probably really want to understand it and when you start searching you will just find lots of scary things. I'm going to send you an academic article about this condition and all of the possible scenarios and what the procedures are and what happens with this kind of thing." And, you know, by the time my daughter was delivered I feel like we have learned this article by heart, but it made it so much easier to talk to the doctors and understand what it is they're talking about.

In saying "no" to the constraints of time and listening to women and spending time helping them understand their conditions, Dr. Fischer not only offered comfort during stressful events but empowered them to have conversations with other medical staff.

Dr. Fischer was not the only medical provider who took the time to listen to mothers and talked with them as partners, but his behavior was consistently celebrated by the women who worked with them in their labors. Other medical staff—including nurses, midwives, and other obstetricians—were similarly appreciated by birth parents for the behaviors exemplified by Dr. Fischer: compassionate and clear communication, active listening, and respectful care. In Lisa's words, "[They] treated us like family."

When medical staff took the time to recognize the feelings mothers might have in the midst of these experiences, women found it to be empowering and meaningful. For example, Beth recalls when a colleague of Dr. Fischer, Dr. Miller, took an extra step to be vulnerable, ask for consent, and recognize her experience,

> They were trying to get me on to the operating table and then Dr. Miller came into the picture and, I feel like time just kind of stood still. He just kind of stopped. He was very calm, he just got everyone to stop and he's like, "she hasn't even consented to surgery yet. It needs to be her decision" . . . [After the surgery] Dr. Miller came in and he was just like, "I'm so sorry that this is how your birth ended up and you didn't get what you wanted." And he's like, "I wish I had more time to talk you through what we are doing, you made the right decision . . . " He was kinda our rock through that.

Women particularly celebrated the times when medical staff respected them enough to trust their intuition about their bodies. Samantha, for example, recalls approaching Dr. Fischer with a feeling that something was wrong,

> I was really sad, and I was crying all the time and I didn't know why. I was really tired, so I went to see Dr. Fischer. I think it was just a regular appointment . . . this is when I decided that I love this man. And I'm like in his office in Greenfield and I'm trying to talk to him about how I was more-than-pregnancy sad . . . and he was so good about it. He didn't dismiss me. He trusted me and said, "Ok let's test a couple of things."

Mothers also found comfort and healing in what they saw as medical staff going beyond their duty to provide kindness and care. For example, Meghan recalls a nurse helping her acquire food vouchers and a room at the Ronald McDonald House when her son was transferred to a larger, urban hospital. Samantha reminisces about how much it meant to her that Dr. Fischer stopped by every morning she was hospitalized, even on the weekend. Other women remarked on how touched they were that Dr. Fischer called to check on them during their NICU stay.

In his actions, Dr. Fischer says "no" to the expectations of time and pushes against the power-knowledge system that hurts mothers, creating the possibility of something different, something better. As was explored earlier in this book, Foucault views institutions as controlling those living within its reach through governing their time, routines, and space. People can resist this power by, as sociologist Rahsaan Mahadeo argues, "tak[ing] 'their' time" back from the systems that control them."[6] It is through this taking of time that people not only claim agency and push back against power structures but also facilitate the creation of new knowledge and associated routines. Applied to this case, we see that Dr. Fischer takes time for the women under his care, resisting the system that demands expediency and efficiency while denying women control and care over their bodies. In doing so, he makes room for compassion, empathy, and the sharing of knowledge women need to feel safe and supported during birth.

KNOWLEDGE FROM BELOW

In her 1975 essay, *The Laugh of the Medusa,* feminist philosopher Hélène Cixous calls on women to write and create knowledge.[7] In reflecting on the ways that women's knowledge and voices have been ignored in the production of knowledge, she contends that women can reclaim their bodies, desires, identities, and selves through writing.

Building off this framework, at the end of our interviews, we asked the women we talked with what they would change to improve obstetric care. The answers ranged but generally fell along the themes of time, space, and routine. Though not written (per Cixous), through telling their stories and offering insights, the women we interviewed make visible the injurious nature of the existing obstetric system and produce new knowledge on ways to improve care.

Making Time

Making time was the most common recommendation offered by women, most of whom felt rushed and ignored during their child's birth. Renee suggests that doctors "Make time for them. And to realize that, like, sure this doctor may deliver five babies today. But I may only deliver one baby in my whole life. And, so, it's a very significant time for me. And I just wish that they would see you more as a person."

Women are able to see how time and the lack of time given to them undermine their body autonomy. Nancy, for instance, shares her concerns that women are "pushed" into having "a c-section or to be induced by a certain time" to accommodate the schedule of the doctor. Another participant, Emma, believes doctors need to be taught "more compassion and really listening to what the person has to say and why." She also focuses on time, indicating that medical staff can improve a mother's experience "just being willing to take the time and ask the questions."

By taking time, doctors resist the structural patterns that harm women. They create room for compassion and humanity and restore power to women. In fact, over half of the women we interviewed craved doctors who would "understand your patients are people," in the words of Rhonda. Or, as Renee said, "realize that they're dealing with full, complex people who have anxieties and fears and past drama . . . and view them that way." Samantha speaks to this as well, suggesting that doctors offer "more personal attention to me and my emotional well-being." She hungered for support after her daughter was transferred to the NICU and wishes her doctor had thought to "check in with the mother."

During the labor, itself, many women offered suggestions to improve communication and compassion and elicit the sense of respect they need and deserve. Samantha, for example, suggested hospitals have "a nurse whose job is solely to talk you through your c-section." Similarly, Trish suggests that hospitals should provide doulas for all patients as a free (or insurance-covered) service during every birth. These doulas could help explain procedures or "help women reason through things . . . and help them think through problems."

One of our nonregional participants actually had the arrangement recommended by Samantha. Gail, who experienced an unwanted cesarean following a long and painful labor, was provided with a nurse whose entire role was to walk her through the birth experience. She found great benefit from this care, recalling: "There was a nurse who held my hand . . . I just remember staring at her and knowing that she had my hand and feeling so grateful that it was someone there with me to give me eye contact . . . [The nurse] told me that she was there with the sole purpose of holding my hand. She said that's all I'm here for. I'm here for you . . . She held my hand. She talked me through it to the best of her ability." Gail's experience suggests that such a shift in care could help mitigate trauma for mothers with difficult childbirths.

Beyond choice and compassion, women wanted the time to receive information. They found among the most injurious parts of their birth the times when they didn't have information to understand current events. Renee, for example, says, "I just wish they explained to me what they were doing and that they explained to me the risks or the benefits of literally everything. Like, why did I have to have a c-section. I still don't know why. You know?"

In short, women wanted doctors to take time for them. They wanted doctors to have the mental space needed to connect with them mindfully. They sought freedom to make decisions and they wanted the information necessary to do so. More than anything, women sought a sense of respect from their doctors during what might be one of the most vulnerable experiences in their life. Decision making, information gathering, and respect all take time. They take time away from the structures that require efficiency and profit. In demanding doctors to take time, women are claiming agency.

Changing Space

Beyond a need to restructure time, women also sought changes to space. As discussed in chapter 2, women are harmed by the way the NICU is organized. Here we see women's suggestions for making space more amenable to their needs.

Prior to her son's birth, Hannah had been flown via air ambulance and subsequently delivered her baby in the city. After his birth, he was transferred to the NICU, but she was moved to the "mother baby floor." Hannah shares that being there was "horrible . . . I could hear babies crying throughout the night" but, unlike the mothers of those infants, she could not see her son or support him in his cries. She requested the medical staff consider moving her somewhere less traumatizing and the nurse she spoke with responded by saying "Well, where else would we put you?"

What Hannah points to here is a fairly basic level of consideration. The separation of mothers from their infants in the NICU is already quite traumatizing for mothers. Hearing babies crying or mothers with their infants—especially when they cannot be with theirs—is very difficult. Providing some distance for women would make a significant difference.

Samantha provides another alternative that would also address Hannah's concern. She also felt acute pain at being separated from her daughter in the NICU and suggests American hospitals consider allowing moms to "room in" with their babies. She contends, "There's a hospital in Europe . . . that allows moms with NICU babies to room in with them the whole time. I would've wanted—I mean I think that's best for the kids too." Samantha contextualizes her statement by saying how sad and heartbroken she felt waking up multiple times "in the middle of the night to pump" while her daughter laid alone in an incubator.

In these suggestions, women say "no" and, in doing so, assert recognition of hidden power systems by calling attention to the way space hurt them and their infants. They recognize how the separation of midwifery and obstetric care cause injury and the ways that the layout of the NICU produces harm. In this recognition, they present a simple solution: keep moms and babies together.

Improving Routine

Women push back against both time and space. They also seek to claim agency over the routines or habits built into the healthcare system that cause injury. In doing so, they say "no" to the idea that a system needs to follow routine because of tradition. They claim agency over bureaucracy.

Dee, for example, suggested more extensive consideration of time during and after birth and connected this plea to the routines of care. She argues that women need to receive more time with doctors following a difficult childbirth, "If nurses and midwives and doctors all took the time . . . If we paid those doctors more and those nurses more and they took that time, would our maternal fetal death rates go down and would we have successful deliveries? . . . If you don't have that time, how can you ask all those questions that's going to help you?" Dee believes that if she was provided with greater support following her birth, then her experiences with postpartum depression would have been reduced.

Women further offered suggestions as to how postpartum care could look differently. Samantha, for example, suggests having a "mother baby center" would help women process their experiences. Such places could house events such as "yoga" and "relaxation" classes. Women could share their stories in a formal support group and lean on one another for healing and advice. Kim agrees, "I think just the fact that women want to talk about it so much and there isn't maybe as much of a venue for retelling those stories . . . I think that even could be a really cathartic process for women."

These centers could also be used to accomplish what Kathy and other women suggest: to prepare women for the possibility of a difficult birth. Many women felt taken by surprise that their birth did not go as planned. They yearned to have had an understanding that this was a possibility for them. Kathy suggests that, as a society, we need to "be willing to discuss trauma in birth" because "not sharing that information" is harmful. She says "it would

have been really nice to know that it could go badly."

The other suggestions were beyond institutional-level care and more focused on systemic changes that would benefit women. For example, Melissa pointed to the need to remove money as a barrier for care. She shares how she skipped much of the prenatal care because of the cost and as a result had more significant complications at her child's birth. Melissa had insurance but still feared the expenses,

> I was just nervous about the cost. I mean, we have good insurance but still, there's that amount that's not covered and I was really nervous about running up a huge hospital bill when we'd already have bills for her and like being out of work for three months, and not having as much financial support in a two-income household where one income is really consistent, but the other is based on commission so we really could not do much extra spending when it came to the medical stuff. And like I was healthy and fine, and I thought that everything would be fine, but if I had known more . . .

In rejecting the current routines of both hospital care and insurance-based health care, women show recognition of the invisible systems that cause them injury. They also make visible some of the discursive practices that injured them, such as social conceptions of ideal birth. Finally, in saying "no" they create the potential for something different, perhaps a single-payer system.

Indeed, survey research shows that when doctors take time to provide clear information, communicate effectively and warmly, and generally build positive relationships with mothers, patient satisfaction increases.[8] These relationships also appear to moderate some of the emotional distress resulting from certain events during women's treatment. Upon close consideration, it is clear that what works for women is a revisioning of the social ranking in health care. Rather than recreating systems that place the doctor above the patient in the management of their treatment, women indicate equalizing this power and involving women in their own care improves their experience.

STRUCTURAL FACTORS THAT FACILITATE
HIGH-QUALITY INTERACTIONS WITH
MEDICAL STAFF: FINLAND

One might question if it is even possible to offer widespread health care in a more personal and humane way. While not perfect, Finland offers an example of how health care, in general, and obstetric care, specifically, could be improved.

Finland approaches health care, especially childbirth, from a radically different knowledge system than the United States. Like most European nations, Finland's healthcare system is funded via a single-payer system. Because health care is viewed as a basic human right, it is run by the government as opposed to private industry. This results in very low cost to patients—in fact, there are upper limits on any medical treatment as charged to the patient—and universal access. It is ranked as one of the most egalitarian models globally.[9] Its healthcare system is rated the best in the world.[10]

Finland has a population of approximately 5.5 million people. Washington State is home to approximately 7.6 million people[11] and about 1.8 million people live in Idaho.[12] Like Idaho and Washington, many residents of Finland live in rural areas or are dispersed in a series of small towns.

To manage care for its residents, Finland has organized a three-tier system of care. The first is at the municipal level. Each municipality is charged with providing and organizing care for its residents. For municipalities with very small populations, they may partner with nearby, similarly small communities. This results in most municipal health systems providing coverage for approximately 20,000 residents.[13] This care typically takes the form of small centers where people receive high-quality, personal care from providers in a family care model.[14] The second tier is a broader hospital system. Finland hosts twenty hospital regions each responsible for treating its inhabitants. For treatments requiring specialists, the nation also hosts five university hospitals that manage such care.[15]

This model results in Finland hosting the second highest ratio of nurses to patients in the European Union at 1,460 nurses per 100,000 residents. In Finland, nurses take on more responsibilities than they do in the United States including case management, consultations, and the prescription of medication. The nation has an average of 320 doctors per 100,000 residents.[16] In contrast, American rural communities house 39.8 doctors per 100,000 residents (in urban communities the ratio is 53.3:100,000).[17] Not only are more doctors per patient available in Finland, they work shorter hours. The average general practitioner works 39.7 hours per week in Finland as opposed to 50.64 hours per week for primary care physicians in the United States.[18] All of these factors result in doctors in Finland having more time to spend with patients, increasing the ability to provide high-quality patient-provider interactions.

Health care in Finland is funded through taxation. The money collected funds the National Health Insurance (NHI) system which covers care for residents and under which all medical providers operate. There is a second, employer-based insurance fund but it partners with the NHI in the provision of care. What is most striking is the fact that, even with higher staff to patient ratios and more personalized care, the per capita expenditure on health care in Finland is less than half of the United States at $4,224 per year.[19]

The Finnish approach to neonatal care also differs significantly from the United States. In Finland, medical practitioners emphasize closeness to infants as opposed to solely aiming to improve infant physical heath.[20] As a result of these cultural values, family members—including siblings—are able to stay with infants in the NICU overnight. Infants receive private rooms with beds for family members. Half of these rooms have bathrooms with showers for family. There is also a shared kitchen on each hospital floor. Hospitals also provide laundry services for parents, a shared living room with social events and classes, and a dining room. Each room is equipped with its own refrigerator to store breastmilk.[21]

The ability to stay with their infants would significantly improve the experience for mothers whose babies are in the NICU. For example, take Samantha's experience. Every day she sat by her daughter's side in her shared hospital room and did not know where she would sleep that evening until, ultimately, a room became available in the Ronald McDonald House a half mile away. Once she moved into the Ronald McDonald House, Samantha ended up walking to and from the hospital or taking taxis in order to accommodate her daughter's care times, after having a major surgery.

Rooming-in would not only prevent the stress of having a place to stay and mitigate the need for unhealthy physical exertion after significant surgeries such as cesareans. It would also improve continuity of care for infants and the emotional wellbeing of mothers. Parents in Finland are considered part of the care team. They are integrated into conversations about child health and their emotional relationship to their infant is central to care.

Individual family rooms also enable infants to receive personalized care. Lights, sounds, and activity levels can be organized around an individual infant's needs and abilities. Family members have privacy and may be more comfortable offering skin-to-skin care, talking with their infants, and engaging in other personalized care efforts.[22] In our interview, Samantha recalled experiencing frustration when her daughter was moved to a new room, with a new roommate. This roommate had been in the hospital for a long time, so their family had decorated the entire room and was insistent upon having the radio constantly running for their child. And as long as Samantha's daughter was there, the roommate's family was never present. On the other hand, Samantha's baby required low levels of stimulation. In the end, she had to advocate to have her child moved (again).

As a result of the Finnish structural and cultural approach to obstetric care, the nation has some of the best outcomes for both babies and mothers. For example, Finland has among the lowest rates of both maternal and infant mortality in the world.[23] Finnish babies who receive neonatal care are more likely to be breastfed, which is associated with improved health and wellbeing for infants.[24] The cesarean rate in Finland is about 16 percent (vs. 32% in the United States).[25]

It is important to note the Finnish approach to neonatal care, emphasizing the integration of parents into the care model, is only possible because Finland has a liberal family leave model.[26] In Finland, families are eligible for up to fourteen months paid leave postpartum and a month of leave during pregnancy, funded by nationally provided maternity insurance.[27] In comparison, women in the United States are not guaranteed any paid leave.

Following childbirth, women continue to receive support from the state. Finland is perhaps most famous for its "baby boxes." In 1938, the nation began providing boxes, funded by tax revenue and free for low-income mothers. By 1949, it became available to all parents. These boxes include clothes, sleepsuits, coats, hats, mittens, fingernail clippers, a hairbrush, a thermometer, diapers, bedding, a mattress, toys, books, and much more. The box itself serves as a bassinet.[28]

The Finnish system works. Maternal and infant outcomes in Finland far surpass those of the United States. Maternal mortality, for example, is three out of every 100,000 births in Finland, as compared to 14 per 100,000 in the United States.[29] The infant mortality rate in the United States is 5.3 per 100,000 births as compared to only 2.5 in Finland.[30] While I was unable to find clear rates of postpartum depression in Finland, there is evidence to suggest women in the United States suffer more symptoms of postpartum depression than do women in Europe generally, including Finland.[31] It is worth noting, however, that rates of postpartum depression fail to serve as a good measure of mental health following childbirth and quality of provider-patient interactions. Rates of mental health challenges, such as depression and anxiety, also reflect cultural norms and values around mental health.

Like any institution, however, the Finnish healthcare system reflects local disciplinary power. Perhaps most obvious, in the case of Finland, is the way their system privileges Finnish born, white residents. Immigrants experience discrimination, greater difficulty accessing care, and higher rates of infant and maternal mortality than do white people born in Finland.[32]

STRONG POSTPARTUM MENTAL HEALTH SUPPORT

Finland provides high-quality maternity care for women. They also continue care for mothers following childbirth through supporting paid leave, continued care for infants and mothers, and the famous baby boxes. It is harder, however, to evaluate Finland and other countries' successes in supporting women's mental health following childbirth. What we do know, however, is postnatal mental health support can help women cope with associated mental health struggles. In doing so, it can improve the mother-infant relationship and outcomes for infants.

While there is not a clear global leader in postpartum mental health care, Germany is often regarded as the model for mental health care more broadly given its unique integration of in- and out-patient support, a patient's primary care doctor, and specialists. Like other European nations, Germany has a public healthcare system under which all of an individual's healthcare needs are covered. This includes mental health care. About 86 percent of Germans use this system; the remaining residents purchase private insurance.[33] It is mandatory to have health coverage in Germany.

Despite important practices—universal, free coverage, and the involvement of general practitioners—Germany and nations with similar practices still fail to meet the mental healthcare needs of all residents. According to the Lancet Commission on Global Mental Health, a group sponsored by *The Lancet* journal that seeks to expand and improve mental healthcare throughout the world, only 20 percent of people with depression in wealthy nations are able to access care. Globally, nations fail to provide needed financial support for people with mental illness to access and participate in care. They also fail to fully invest in needed research into mental health and care.[34]

The Lancet Commission on Global Mental Health suggests several strategies to improve care across nations. They suggested more community-based (as opposed to institutionalized) care for people struggling with their mental health. They promote cultural change to avoid stigmas associated with mental illness. They seek to expand societal understandings of mental illness to include various aspects of mental well-being. Finally, they advocate for preventative care—facilitating resilience among people who have not yet dealt with mental health challenges. To do this, the commission sees a need to increase funding for research and support for mental health care.[35]

Despite the lack of a clear model for postpartum mental health support, there are evidence-based practices in other nations that help new mothers. In northern and western European nations, new mothers receive home visits from healthcare professionals following childbirth. In the Netherlands, new mothers are eligible for a free (insurance provided) home care program that includes childcare, care for mothers, and housekeeping.[36] In Norway, women have the option of remaining in the maternity center following birth. This enables families to remain together in a hotel-like environment wherein the mother and newborn continue to be cared for by nursing staff.[37] Regardless of whether this care occurs in the home or at maternity centers, this transitional time empowers women to develop new parenting skills and allows them time to physically heal from giving birth.

CONCLUSION: IMPROVING CARE

Low-quality patient-provider interactions harm mothers who have already experienced a physically traumatic childbirth. In contrast, high-quality interactions, such as those outlined in this chapter, can mitigate some of a woman's traumatic experience. The women we interviewed cited several areas of care that could be improved to prevent or minimize trauma for mothers. Suggestions focus on a reorganization of time, space, and routine and include more time spent between physicians and mothers, allowing women to room-in with their babies in the NICU, providing better communication to mothers, perhaps through a nurse or doula whose sole job is to talk a mother through events and improving access to much needed postnatal care.

As we covered in chapter 1, the current model of obstetric care in the United States emerges from the nation's own systems of knowledge. Fear of a powerful centralized government led, instead, to the corrupt control of for-profit insurance industries. The associated drive to increase profits results in staffing shortages and high demands on doctors to see patients quickly. This pressure decreases their ability to provide high-quality care for mothers. Finland, in contrast, emerged from its own systems of knowledge and created a fully funded, more family-centered care system. Germany, too, provides a more integrated approach to mental health care that could reduce mothers' suffering.

While institutions operate from their fundamental system of knowledge, they are not total in their control. Rather, people within the system have the power to create alternative knowledge and challenge existing systems. We see this process in the actions of doctors such as Dr. Fischer who say "no" to limiting temporal structures and, instead, take time with mothers pushing against the norms within obstetric care.

NOTES

1. Kevin Jon Heller, "Power, subjectification and resistance in Foucault," *SubStance* 25, no. 1 (1996): 78–110.

2. Susan Bordo, "Feminism, Foucault, and the politics of the body," in *Bodies and Pleasures,* edited by Ladelle McWhorter, 179–201. Bloomington, IN: Indiana University Press, 1999.

3. Susan Bordo, *Unbearable Weight* (Berkley, CA: University of California Press, 2004), 27.

4. Sara Ahmed, "No" Accessed February 28, 2021, https://feministkilljoys.com/2 017/06/30/no/.

5. Naykky Singh Ospina, Kari A. Phillips, Rene Rodriguez-Gutierrez, Ana Castaneda-Guarderas, Michael R. Gionfriddo, Megan E. Branda, and Victor M. Montori, "Eliciting the patient's agenda-secondary analysis of recorded clinical encounters," *Journal of General Internal Medicine* 34, no. 1 (2019): 36–40.

6. Rahsaan Mahadeo, "Funk the clock: Transgressing time while young, prescient and black," (2019).

7. Hélène Cixous, "The laugh of the Medusa," *Signs* 1, no. 4 (1976).

8. Sheera F. Lerman, Golan Shahar, Kathryn A. Czarkowski, Naamit Kurshan, Urania Magriples, Linda C. Mayes, and C. Neill Epperson, "Predictors of satisfaction with obstetric care in high-risk pregnancy: The importance of patient–provider relationship," *Journal of Clinical Psychology in Medical Settings* 14, no. 4 (2007): 330–334.

9. Emily Tamkin, "Finland's health-care system is ranked among the best in the world. Someone Tell Nikki Haley," *The Washington Post.* March 21, 2019. Accessed June 6, 2020. https://www.washingtonpost.com/world/2019/03/21/finlands-health-c are-system-is-ranked-among-best-world-someone-tell-nikki-haley/.

10. Sintia Radu, "Countries with the most well-developed health care systems," *U.S. News and World Report.* January 21, 2020. Accessed July 6, 2020. https://www .usnews.com/news/best-countries/slideshows/countries-with-the-most-well-develop ed-public-health-care-system?onepage.

11. United States Census Bureau, 2019, "Quickfacts: Washington," Accessed June 20, 2020. https://www.census.gov/quickfacts/WA.

12. United States Census Bureau, 2019, "Quickfacts: Idaho," Accessed June 20, 2020. https://www.census.gov/quickfacts/fact/table/ID/PST045219.

13. Dionne S. Kringos, Wienke GW Boerma, Allen Hutchinson, and Richard B. Saltman, *Building Primary Care in a Changing Europe. Case Studies.* WHO Regional Office for Europe, 2015.

14. Finnish Medical Association, "Overview of the healthcare system in Finland," *Health Management* 7, no. 5 (2007). https://healthmanagement.org/c/imaging/issuea rticle/overview-of-the-healthcare-system-in-finland.

15. Finnish Medical Association, "Overview of the Healthcare System in Finland."

16. OECD/European Observatory on Health Systems and Policies, 2017, "State of the Health of the EU: Finland," OECD Publishing. Paris/European Observatory on Health Systems and Policies, Brussels. http://dx.doi.org/10.1787/978926428 3367-en.

17. National Rural Health Association, "About rural health care," Accessed August 20, 2020. https://www.ruralhealthweb.org/about-nrha/about-rural-health-care.

18. The Physicians Foundation, "2018 Survey of America's Physicians." The Physicians Foundation. Accessed August 20, 2020. https://physiciansfoundation.org/wp-content/uploads/2018/09/physicians-survey-results-final-2018.pdf.

19. Organization for Economic Co-operation and Development, 2020, "Health Spending." Accessed June 20, 2020. https://data.oecd.org/healthres/health-spending.htm.

20. Sarah Holdren, Cynthia Fair, and Liisa Lehtonen, "A qualitative cross-cultural analysis of NICU care culture and infant feeding in Finland and the US," *BMC Pregnancy and Childbirth* 19, no. 1 (2019): 1–12.

21. Holdren et al., "A qualitative cross-cultural analysis of NICU care," 345.

22. Robert D. White, "Individual rooms in the NICU—an evolving concept," *Journal of Perinatology* 23, no. 1 (2003): S22–S24.

23. Marian F. MacDorman, T. J. Mathews, Ashna D. Mohangoo, and Jennifer Zeitlin, "International comparisons of infant mortality and related factors: United States and Europe, 2010." (2014).

24. Holdren et al., "A qualitative cross-cultural analysis of NICU care," 345.

25. Center for Disease Control, "Births—method of delivery," Accessed September 3, 2020. https://www.cdc.gov/nchs/fastats/delivery.htm; Pyykönen, Aura, Mika Gissler, Ellen Løkkegaard, Thomas Bergholt, Steen C. Rasmussen, Alexander Smárason, Ragnheiður I. Bjarnadóttir et al., "Cesarean section trends in the Nordic Countries–a comparative analysis with the Robson classification," *Acta obstetricia et gynecologica Scandinavica* 96, no. 5 (2017): 607–616.

26. Holdren et al., "A qualitative cross-cultural analysis of NICU care," 345.

27. Marja-Terttu Tarkka, Marita Paunonen, and Pekka Laippala, "Social support provided by public health nurses and the coping of first-time mothers with child care," *Public Health Nursing* 16, no. 2 (1999): 114–119; Laurel Wamsley, "Finland's women-led government had equalized family leave," February 5, 2020. Accessed February 13, 2021. https://www.npr.org/2020/02/05/803051237/finlands-women-led-government-has-equalized-family-leave-7-months-for-each-parent.

28. Helena Lee, "Why Finnish babies sleep in cardboard boxes," *BBC News.* June 4, 2013. Accessed November 1, 2020. https://www.bbc.com/news/magazine-22751415.

29. Central Intelligence Agency, 2015, "Country comparisons: Maternal mortality rate" The World Factbook. Accessed November 8, 2020. https://www.cia.gov/library/publications/the-world-factbook/rankorder/2223rank.html.

30. Central Intelligence Agency, 2015, "Country comparisons: Infant mortality rate," The World Factbook. Accessed November 8, 2020 https://www.cia.gov/library/Publications/the-world-factbook/fields/354rank.html.

31. Dyanne D. Affonso, Anindya K. De, June Andrews Horowitz, and Linda J. Mayberry, "An international study exploring levels of postpartum depressive symptomatology," *Journal of Psychosomatic Research* 49, no. 3 (2000): 207–216.

32. Laura Kemppainen, Teemu Kemppainen, Natalia Skogberg, Hannamaria Kuusio, and Päivikki Koponen, "Immigrants 'use of health care in their country of origin: the role of social integration, discrimination and the parallel use of health care systems," *Scandinavian Journal of Caring Sciences* 32, no. 2 (2018): 698–706; Maili

Malin, and Mika Gissler, "Maternal care and birth outcomes among ethnic minority women in Finland," *BMC Public Health* 9, no. 1 (2009), doi:10.1186/1471-2458-9-84.

33. Having insurance in Germany is mandatory. Therefore, if one turns down the public insurance option, they must purchase private insurance. Sarah Fielding, "What America can learn from the mental health care systems of other countries," *Talk Space*. April 6, 2020. Accessed November 8, 2020. https://www.talkspace.com/blog/america-mental-health-care-systems/.

34. Joanne Silberner, "Report: World support for mental health care is 'pitifully small,'" *NPR*. October 15, 2018. Accessed November 8, 2020. https://www.npr.org/sections/goatsandsoda/2018/10/15/656669752/report-world-support-for-mental-health-care-is-pitifully-small.

35. Silberner, "Report: World support for mental health care is 'pitifully small.'"

36. Ching-Yu Cheng, Eileen R. Fowles, and Lorraine O. Walker, "Postpartum maternal health care in the United States: A critical review," *The Journal of Perinatal Education* 15, no. 3 (2006): 34; De Vries, Raymond, Cecilia Benoit, Edwin Van Teijlingen, and Sirpa Wrede, eds. *Birth by Design: Pregnancy, Maternity Care and Midwifery in North America and Europe* (Routledge, 2002).

37. Cheng et al., "Continuing education module," 34–42.

Conclusion

Changing Knowledge

Through the pages of this book, I identified and analyzed institutional structures and ideologies that cause or exacerbate mothers' injury during childbirth.
The women we talked with felt traumatized as a result of the actual events
they endured (emergency cesareans, stillbirth, etc.), but they also experienced
trauma—or deepened trauma—as a result of poor interactions with medical
providers. Women were injured by absent communication from medical
practitioners—times when they did not know the status of themselves or their
infants. They felt harmed when they faced intervention without consent, also
known as obstetric violence. Medical practitioners further hurt mothers when
they acted in a disrespectful manner, through their words or actions, such as
by engaging in microaggressions or using offensive language.

Poor interactions between providers and mothers result from the restrictions placed on medical staff within the U.S. healthcare system as a result of
the ideologies upon which it was built (power-knowledge systems). These
ideologies (or power-knowledge) discipline practitioners and women through
exerting control over their time, space, and routine.

Medical practitioners work extraordinary hours and have limited *time* with
patients. These forces combine and cause mental, physical, and emotional
stress for medical staff, which can manifest in poor interactions with patients
as well as medical accidents. Long hours result in part from staffing shortages
that plague the nation as a whole, but especially rural healthcare systems.

Women are controlled by *space*. The artificial segregation of midwifery
from obstetrics harms women who have to traverse the two. Women with
babies who need NICU care are injured not only by the agonizing stress of
worrying about their sick baby but also struggle with the structure of the
space and the unnatural distance from their babies.

Finally, women are controlled by *routine*. Women who live in rural areas are disproportionately unemployed, working class, and reliant on Medicaid. They have to travel greater distances to access obstetric care and even then may be unable to find high-level care needed for women with high-risk pregnancies. As a result, rural mothers are also harmed by other structural factors, particularly practices associated with Medicaid. Medicaid disproportionately rejects coverage for certain needed interventions. Women also face stigma from doctors who perceive or treat Medicaid patients as a second tier of clients. Routine, too, contributes to the relatively high rates of infant and maternal mortality in the United States.

These structures reflect and are supported by underlying knowledge systems that also exacerbate trauma for women directly. We see glimpses of this knowledge in the ways it privileges fetal rights over women's. We witness misogynistic norms used to justify the mistreatment of patients, particularly women of color and low-income women. We also perceive how these ideologies are internalized by women in ways that cause internal turmoil and problems in their relationships.

Finally, in chapter 7, we saw the way doctors and women can take time, space, and routine away from the systems that harm them to demand a more humane system of care. While still an institution, certain countries, such as Finland and Germany, offer possibilities for improvements to our own.

POSSIBILITIES FOR CHANGE

To make these changes, we need to alter the system of knowledge upon which our healthcare system operates. While this sounds insurmountable, we see evidence of past successes. Early obstetric care did little to mitigate women's pain during childbirth. Even cesarean sections were performed without anesthesia. This is unheard of in the present. Throughout the twentieth century, the United States routinely sterilized women without their consent. While this practice still happens today, it occurs less as an accepted form of obstetric care, instead hiding in the shadows only visible in glimpses through limited, typically critical media attention.

According to Foucault, social change happens when systems of knowledge are altered. Power is a tool used to generate knowledge, and thereby change the accepted norms and discourse of a society. When people like Dr. Fischer take time and give it to women, this pushes back against the coercive system. When women tell the stories of their traumatic births, it rejects the status quo and resists this injurious system of knowledge. In these instances, they are changing knowledge.

The women we interviewed have keen insight into the way the current system fails and, as such, also produce important knowledge for its alteration. In what follows, I present a simplified list of the suggestions offered by both the women we interviewed and the possibilities presented by the practices in Finland, Germany, and other nations (see chapter 7).

First and fundamentally, the United States needs to provide free, universal health coverage that includes mental health care. This will eliminate the financial barrier to support cited by many of the women we interviewed and improve mothers' mental health and prevent negative impacts on infants. The universal healthcare model will also allow for increased staffing and reduced pressure on medical practitioners as is evident in comparing U.S. care to that of other nations.

Second, the United States needs to provide extended, paid leave for parents preceding and following a child's birth.[1] It needs to give women time. Paid leave helps women heal physically and mentally from childbirth. Women who take leave have lower rates of depression and greater levels of health than those who are unable to do so. Women whose partners take leave also report higher levels of mental health than those who do not.[2] As discussed in chapter 6, women who are able to take leave are financially better off than women who are forced back to work soon after their child's birth. The provision of paid leave is a significant equity issue, allowing low-income women the same right to physical and mental health, without concern for their family's economic wellbeing during this time. Family leave also enables mothers to succeed in other important aspects of maternal care. For example, paid leave is associated with higher rates of breastfeeding for mothers, which provides physical and emotional benefits to both mother and child.[3]

Third, the United States needs to revolutionize the current approach to NICU care. The present setup is harmful to women and their infants as they are separated from one another at an important time of bonding and care. Adopting a family-centered approach like that of Finland provides a more heart- and compassion-centered framework of care that benefits all parties involved. It involves family members in infant's care and keeps the family unit together in a comfortable space, setting them up for success upon the infant's departure from the NICU.

Fourth, the United States needs an integrated healthcare model (also called collaborative care model) that involves and connects a woman's general practitioner, obstetrician, midwife, and local mental health specialists in a mother's pre-natal, obstetric, and postpartum care. We must further welcome midwifery and doula care into hospitals nationwide and normalize out-of-hospital births. These changes will ease the burdens of space and routine for mothers. Collaborative care has been shown to provide better coordination and management of care for patients, to have superior monitoring and treatment and better care for those who do not respond to initial treatment.[4] They also cost less.[5] Psychologists, counselors, primary care physicians, and patients alike have expressed support for these programs.

Fifth, we need a shift in public discourse surrounding postnatal mental health that reduces its stigma and normalizes mental health care. The Mayo Clinic suggests that current social stigmas around mental health prevent people from accessing care, limit the support people struggling with mental health experience, can impact patients' job and housing prospects, may prevent insurance from covering needed care, and further harm patients' self-worth.[6] While the aforementioned collaborative care approach does not change mental health stigmas across American culture, it does enable patients to avoid much of the shame and negative repercussions mentioned above.

Finally, the United States should invest in the provision of free community support opportunities for new mothers. These services could be support groups for women who survived traumatic births or simply places for women to go and connect or seek practical advice for their new roles as mothers. Examples of efficacious support groups are those designed for pregnant women who have previously lost children via stillbirth or later death. These groups have successfully helped women connect to others with similar experiences, process their fears, protect the memories of their children who have passed, and to develop important skills to cope.[7] Some women also benefit from virtual opportunities to connect with other moms. Research suggests that Facebook mom and pregnancy groups can provide important social support for women, help reduce stress, and provide practical advice.[8] To connect this back to the specific case of traumatic birth, it is clear that telling one's story can alleviate trauma.[9] Whether that happens in a support group, a one-on-one conversation with a therapist, or in online spaces may matter less than the act of sharing one's experience itself. The process of storytelling can help women process their experience but also claim ownership and find empowerment redefining trauma as survivorship.[10]

To make these structural changes, there needs to be a corresponding alteration in the broader power/knowledge system—the ideological realities that construct and shape institutions. I end this manuscript, then, by exploring how discursive change happens.

HOW SOCIAL CHANGE HAPPENS

Through this book I have used Foucault's concept of biopower and associated ideas of power-knowledge and discipline as a scaffolding for understanding the operation of obstetric care and the ways it causes injury, pain, and trauma to mothers. In chapter 7, I extended his analysis of social change by drawing on the work of feminist thinkers. To end, I further this analysis, drawing from the crucial work of feminist philosophers Susan Bordo, Judith Butler, and Sara Ahmed.

Within a given society, there are concurrent, competing knowledge systems. Even a dominant knowledge system in a given society operates parallel to others. Consider, for example, social beliefs regarding same-sex marriage. From a Foucauldian analysis, we see how historical knowledge prioritizing heterosexuality serves as the foundation for U.S. institutions. Queer people were excluded from marriage, adoption, and other civil practices due to the institutional patterns reinforcing heterosupremacy. People were driven into the metaphorical "closet" through the internalization of this knowledge system and associated self-sanctioning and disciplining. Throughout U.S. history, queer people were imprisoned, arrested, or even sterilized to reinforce this knowledge system. Yet, in recent years, a parallel, subversive ideological framework, one that values equity and rejects the supremacy of heterosexuality has risen. It rose through fissures within the knowledge-system of heterosupremacy to the extent that many blatant, discriminatory laws have changed. Same-sex marriage is now legal nationwide. Many (but not all) states have legalized same-sex adoption. To be clear, I am not saying that the fight for queer rights is over. Rather, I employ this example to show an active, current example of how knowledge systems are disrupted by the actions of those who dissent.

From Foucault, then, we see that knowledge systems are not absolute. They have fissures or, as Sara Ahmed describes it, leaks and spills.[11] These fissures can be capitalized upon by people to both resist existing norms and values (and their patterning in social structures) and also for the creation of new knowledge systems. Yet, despite his profound attention to power, Foucault fails to offer a clear analysis of resistance or change to power/ knowledge systems.[12]

Poststructural feminism more broadly provides insight into how resistance can alter existing discourses and knowledge. Philosopher Susan Bordo, for example, in her book *Unbearable Weight*, examines the cultural context through which the practices of anorexia and bulimia emerge. In this work, she extends Foucault's consideration of social change and contends that "dominant forms and institutions are continually being penetrated and reconstructed by values, styles, and knowledges that have been developing and gathering strength, energy and distinctiveness 'at the margins.'"[13] Bordo argues further that such change is neither instantly radical nor revolutionary in its alteration, but slow. She suggests, "Such transformations do not occur in one fell swoop; they emerge only gradually, through local and often minute shifts in power."[14]

What, then, do these "minute" but constant changes look like? According to philosopher Sara Ahmed, they often look like "complaints" or saying "no."

Ahmed argues in her forthcoming book *Complaint!* and throughout her blog, *Feminist Killjoys*, that complaining is a method of pushing against power structures. It first serves to make visible power systems as they operate, but also warns those who may encounter such systems in the future, all while pushing against and challenges these structures.[15]

In this work, Ahmed draws on that of feminist philosopher Judith Butler. In Butler's writing on gender, she demonstrates how power creates humans as subjects. Furthermore, in rejecting power in its existing form, individuals (in the case of obstetric care, medical staff and mothers) say "I am not going to be subjected in this way or by these means through which the state establishes its legitimacy."[16] Thus, saying "no" not only rejects the ideological status quo but also the subjugation of those within its influence.

Such acts of resistance—complaints, saying no—are not without risk. Ahmed writes extensively about the reactions to complaints and points to, among other challenges, the ways that saying no inspires others to increase violence against the naysayer. In her blog, she uses the example of refusing to laugh at a sexist joke—saying no to misogynistic humor. In response, Ahmed argues, you become "known as a feminist" and "violence is channeled in your direction."[17] This is true, perhaps even more so, in response to the lodging of formal complaints.

Knowledge systems, then, change in response to the production of counter-narratives, saying no and making complaints. Such alternative knowledges can exploit the fissures and weaknesses within oppressive systems. Social change happens via the concurrent shifts in both systems of knowledge and associated change in social systems. If we can think of completing knowledges as operating on different levels, as determined by their reach, we see that (at least in the United States) certain knowledges dominate the operation of most social structures and control of human thoughts and actions. These include capitalism (and the associated myths of meritocracy), white supremacy, and misogyny, among others. Capitalism, in particular, is so ingrained in the way people think and act in U.S. society as to be invisible in its control.

In the case of traumatic births, American values that reject a strong federal government and concurrent privileging of the ideas of free-market capitalism have led to the construction of an insurance-based model of care. In its efforts toward efficiency, health care has thus become an inhumane system (an Iron Cage, in Weberian parlance) controlling and coercing doctors, staff, and patients. Doctors are tasked with seeing multiple patients quickly, limiting their ability to provide high-quality interactions with patients. Moreover, the institution itself was built on unjust knowledge systems (i.e., misogyny, white supremacy, and capitalism). Thus, by behaving in ways they feel are "natural" or routine, doctors reinforce systems that hurt patients.

How, then, can we change both the structures and knowledge systems of American health care? In this context, too, we have a particular challenge in the creation of alternative knowledge systems. The political right in the United States has secured great power over public discourse and, through defunding public schools, they have essentially undermined the systems from which those able to see through the invisible walls of power/knowledge will rise. The war of ideas is ongoing, but both the political right has significant strength in this politically divided nation. In fact, they have successfully relied heavily on a disinformation campaign to push back against the possibility of universal health care.[18]

Drawing on these theorists, my vision for social change is as follows. First, we need to listen to and amplify the voices of women. While Cixous contends women's agency can be reclaimed through writing their stories, oral narratives such as that presented here further employs and engages with power. In other words, those existing in and hurt by the current knowledge system need to exploit the existing fissures as often as possible, even in localized ways through interrupting and altering social discourse that sees the current system as natural and inevitable. These efforts need to be bolstered through the complaints made by others, both warning mothers yet to give birth and to push against institutional coercion and control.

I'd like to pause here to briefly point to a fallacy I see in ideas surrounding social change. Many contend neo-liberalism has driven us to look at only individual action as it relates to social change.[19] So, for example, we talk about solving the climate crisis through individual actions to reduce a household's carbon footprint. They contend, instead, that focus needs to be on changing systems, such as industrial agriculture. I fear that such a framework provides an excuse for inaction that prevents effective collective action. In truth, both of these processes need to occur. It is through individual change, and discussion of that change, that discourses shift and new knowledge systems are produced. It is through the changing in discourse that what is acceptable behavior is altered. The national conversations about reducing one's carbon footprint, for example, motivate collective action based on what is acceptable carbon production. People are, in effect, shamed into being more eco-friendly.

In my classes, I talk to my students about the process of social change. Drawing on poststructuralist thought, I contend, as does Bordo, that discursive alterations happen constantly and consistently in small ways. That, in any given moment, in any behavior, action, inaction, or interaction, we either reproduce existing power/knowledge systems or reject and recreate them—perhaps subtly, perhaps more robustly.

I give the following examples from a single evening in my own life, of times I both failed to challenge dominant discourse and times I resisted. While in graduate school, I played on a team in a gay softball league. My team attended a tournament in Milwaukee. After a day of playing, we went to a nightclub. Hungry, I walked across the street to purchase food from a gas station. When I walked in, I observed a long line of customers waiting behind a frantic man begging for the attendant to let him put $0.50 of gas in his tank. The attendant was unable to do so; he said, the system would not allow purchases in such small amounts. As the line behind him groaned, the man became increasingly upset. In that moment, I had a choice. I could do nothing and allow our ideological systems surrounding the shame and disgust toward people in poverty to persist, or I could disrupt the discourse. I walked to the man and handed him a five-dollar bill so he could get gas. I said no to the existing ideological structure, both making it visible and giving permission to others to do the same.

However, on my way out of the store, I failed to repeat this resistance in the face of another oppressive knowledge system. As I waited in line to pay, now with only one person ahead of me, I heard the man at the front of the line make disparaging remarks regarding a person in drag pumping gas outside. He looked at me with a leer, expecting my laugh and consent to his reproduction of heterosupremacist and misogynistic knowledge systems. While I did not offer him consent, I failed to say "no." I ignored him and permitted these oppressive forces to reproduce.

Our life is riddled with these moments. Moments when we can through our action or inaction reproduce or reinforce existing power/knowledge systems. Or, we can say "no." We can complain and contribute to producing a new knowledge. These moments may be discursive, as the examples I produced above, or they could be actions aimed at changing policy.

In her work, Ahmed talks extensively about her and others' work on improving equity. She contends in her blog that "in order to survive institutions, we need to transform them" and offers as one strategy, what she calls "complaint collectives."[20] Institutions will resist change, Ahmed argues, but as each complaint is made, it is "picked up and amplified by others." It expands and gains traction and force.

It is by capitalizing on this traction and bolstering complaint collectives that we can alter institutional policies. For example, 2020 brought a wave of protests against anti-Black police violence in the United States. These protests are an example of collectives of people saying "no" to continued institutionally sanctioned murder. Though violently shut down in individual locations, the power of this "no" grew such that throughout the country cities began to question their policing policies and universities have been further called upon to examine equity in their own institutions.[21]

As predicted by Ahmed, BLM protests and even higher education efforts have been met by violence. In the case of protests, this has been largely overt physical and institutional violent control. In the case of higher education, this has been through concerted right-wing efforts to dismantle progress toward equity in colleges and universities.[22]

Perhaps a better explanation comes from Ibram Kendi's book *How to Be an Anti-Racist* in which Kendi argues that any thought, behavior, or policy is either anti-racist or racist, in that it upholds the status quo. There are no race-neutral policies, he contends, because race neutrality upholds the narratives and power structures that advantage white people. Change then happens, offers Kendi, when collectives acknowledge and identify racism and racist policy, develop and implement antiracist policy and drive associated discourse in partnership with allies, and to monitor the successes or failures of newly implemented policies.

Replacing the power/knowledge system that produces and maintains the current system of obstetric care will not be easy. Change of this magnitude requires sustained efforts at saying "no," to identify the current invisible power operations, to warn others, and to push against them. We need to listen to the stories of women who have survived, to hear their insights and solutions as we work to resist and change power system. Through the complication of minute attempts into "complaint collectives" we produce counter knowledge systems and maintain the momentum needed to shift discourse accordingly. As these fissures or "spills" expand, we gain the ability to implement better and equitable policies, changing the institutional manifestation of power/knowledge in new ways.

FINAL THOUGHTS

It is not my goal in this book to villainize medical professionals nor blame women for their pain. Quite the contrary. I think both of these parties strive to do the best they can within a system that exerts powerful controls over their thoughts and actions. Both groups are truly heroic. My aim, then, is to help explain the institutional and ideological practices that hurt women. It is not individuals who are at fault for this system; it is the very structure itself. The history of our society as it seeps into the present day. This legacy as it ventures forth, peaking out at us through identifiable patterns of pain and trauma.

The United States is rooted in an ideology of white supremacy, meritocracy, and misogyny. These systems of power were built into our social structure, including health care. We recognize it in how women in the United States are disproportionately harmed during obstetric care. It is visible in the way women of color and poor women make up the majority of people suffering and dying during childbirth.

The obstetric care system in the United States is not natural. It does not need to continue in its current form. While Finland offers one model for how health care can be offered in a less oppressive but still imperfect way, it is not the only possibility. I suggest, instead, we listen to those most harmed by the current system to build one anew. The women I interviewed had clear suggestions of ways to improve maternal health care. These incremental steps would help reduce the suffering of many women within the obstetric care system. However, for real change to happen, there needs to be a broader "complaint collective" (amplified by individual actions to say "no" and change discourse in everyday life) toward free universal health care in the United States.

To change the current system, we must listen to the women who have survived it. We need to embrace the knowledge their embodied experiences produce and use them to reform existing structures. Such action requires that we complain loudly, consistently, and collectively. As Ahmed contends, complaining will not only provide greater insight into the power systems as they operate but will also serve to warn new mothers and concurrently make visible and slowly change existing practices. Only through making the invisible operation of power/knowledge visible will we adequately change the knowledge systems that constrain us. We must work to resist the current model by exploiting its fissures and challenging its normalcy at every opportunity.

In many ways, this book seeks to be a resounding no—a complaint to make visible existing power systems, warn women of its harm, and push back—joining the voices of many others in an attempt to amplify their voices and continue to build momentum toward change.

NOTES

1. Ellen Mozurkewich, "Working conditions and pregnancy outcomes: An updated appraisal of the evidence," *American Journal of Obstetrics & Gynecology*, 222, no. 3 (2020): 201–203.

2. Pinka Chatterji and Sara Markowitz, *Family Leave after Childbirth and the Health of New Mothers*. No. w14156. National Bureau of Economic Research, 2008.

3. Kelsey R. Mirkovic, Cria G. Perrine, Kelley S. Scanlon, and Laurence M. Grummer-Strawn, "Maternity leave duration and full-time/part-time work status are associated with US mothers' ability to meet breastfeeding intentions," *Journal of Human Lactation* 30, no. 4 (2014): 416–419.

4. Jürgen Unützer, Henry Harbin, Michael Schoenbaum, and Benjamin Druss, "The collaborative care model: An approach for integrating physical and mental health care in Medicaid health homes," Advancing Integrated Mental Health Solutions, University of Washington. Accessed November 8, 2020. https://aims.uw .edu/sites/default/files/CMSBrief_2013.pdf.

5. Unützer et al., "The collaborative care model."

6. The Mayo Clinic, 2020, "Mental health: Overcoming the stigma of mental illness," Accessed November 8, 2020. https://www.mayoclinic.org/diseases-conditions /mental-illness/in-depth/mental-health/art-20046477.

7. Denise Côté-Arsenault and Marsha Mason Freije, "Support groups help women through pregnancies after loss," *Western Journal of Nursing Research* 26, no. 6 (2004): DOI: 10.1177/0193945904265817.

8. Bree Holtz, Andrew Smock and David Reyes-Gastelum, "Connected motherhood: Social support for moms and moms-to-be on Facebook," *Telemedicine and e-Health*. 21, no. 5 (2015). https://www.liebertpub.com/doi/abs/10.1089/tmj.2014 .0118.

9. Laurel J. Kiser, Barbara Baumgardner, and Joyce Dorado, "Who are we, but for the stories we tell: Family stories and healing," *Psychological Trauma: Theory, Research, Practice, and Policy* 2, no. 3 (2010): 243; Rachel N. Spear, "'Let Me Tell You a Story' On Teaching Trauma Narratives, Writing, and Healing," *Pedagogy: Critical Approaches to Teaching Literature, Language, Composition, and Culture* 14, no. 1 (2014): 53–79.

10. Brianna C. Delker, Rowan Salton, and Kate C. McLean, "Giving voice to silence: Empowerment and disempowerment in the developmental shift from trauma 'victim' to 'survivor-advocate'," *Journal of Trauma & Dissociation* 21, no. 2 (2020): 242–263.

11. Sara Ahmed, "Feminists at Work," Feminist Killjoys. Accessed February 20, 2021. https://feministkilljoys.com/2020/01/10/feminists-at-work/.

12. Jana Sawicki, "Feminism and the power of discourse," in *After Foucault: Humanistic Knowledge, Postmodern Challenges*, edited by Jonathan Arac (New Brunswick and London: Rutgers University Press, 1988), 161–178.

13. Susan Bordo, *Unbearable Weight* (Berkley, CA: University of California Press, 2004), 27–28.

14. Susan Bordo, *Unbearable Weight* (Berkley, CA: University of California Press, 2004).

15. Sara Ahmed, *Complaint!* (Duke University Press, 2021); Sara Ahmed, "Why Complain?" Feminist Killjoys. Accessed February 20, 2021. http://feministkilljoys.c om/2019/07/22/why-complain.

16. Judith Butler, Interview, Centre de Cultura Contemporània de Barcelona. February 2008. Published in *The Monthly Review*.

17. Sara Ahmed, "No," *Feminist Killjoys*. Accessed February 20, 2021. https://fe ministkilljoys.com/2017/06/30/no/.

18. Sheena Goodyear, "This former U.S. health insurance exec says he lied to Americans about Canadian health care," *As it Happens, Canadian Broadcast Corporation*. June 29, 2020. Accessed November 22, 2020: https://www.cbc.ca/ radio/asithappens/as-it-happens-monday-edition-1.5631285/this-former-u-s-health-i nsurance-exec-says-he-lied-to-americans-about-canadian-health-care-1.5631874.

19. Martin Lukas, "Neoliberalism has conned us into fighting climate change as individuals," *The Guardian*. July 17, 2017. https://www.theguardian.com/environ ment/true-north/2017/jul/17/neoliberalism-has-conned-us-into-fighting-climate-ch ange-as-individuals.

20. Sara Ahmed, "Feminists at Work." Accessed February 20, 2021. https://fe ministkilljoys.com/2020/01/10/feminists-at-work/.

21. Jemima McEvoy, "At least 13 cities are defunding their police departments," *Forbes.* August 12th, 2020. Accessed February 20, 2021. https://www.forbes.com/ sites/jemimamcevoy/2020/08/13/at-least-13-cities-are-defunding-their-police-depart ments/?sh=334ded4829e3; Lindsay McKenzie, "Words matter for college presidents, but so will actions," *Inside Higher Education.* June 8, 2020. Accessed February 20, 2020. https://www.insidehighered.com/news/2020/06/08/searching-meaningful -response-college-leaders-killing-george-floyd; Sydney Freeman, Jr., "10 Concrete policy changes PWIs can enact to show Black lives matter," *Diverse Issues in Higher Education,* June 25, 2020. Accessed February 20, 2021. https://diverseeducation.com /article/182222/.

22. Kevin Richert, "Analysis: Previewing Idaho's next higher education budget battle," *Idaho Education News.* January 28, 2020. Accessed February 20, 2020. https ://www.idahoednews.org/top-news/analysis-previewing-idahos-next-higher-educa tion-budget-battle/.

Appendix A

List of Participants Featured in Book

Participant Name	Location of Birth	Transfer?	NICU Stay?	Other Complications	"Type" of Birth	Race*	Medicaid?**	Additional Children? (As of time of interview)
Alice	North Hospital	Birth center to hospital (prior to birth)	No	Fetal distress, emergency c-section	Cesarean	W	No	No
Lisa	Urban hospital	North Hospital to urban hospital (prior to birth)	Yes	Preeclampsia, pre-term birth, emergency c-section	Cesarean	W	No	No
Jen	North Hospital	No	No	Breech baby, c-section, long labor	Cesarean	W	No	1 following BT
Beth	North Hospital	Birth center to hospital (prior to birth)	No	Breech baby, c-section	Cesarean	W	No	No
Erica	North Hospital	Birth center to hospital (prior to birth)	No	Obstetric violence, infant distress	Vaginal	W	No	1 following BT
Meghan (two traumatic births)	South Hospital	South Hospital to urban hospital (for infant)	Yes	Hyperemesis gravidarum, pre-term birth, bleeding, emergency c-section	Cesarean	W	No	No
Emma	South Hospital	No	No	Pre-term birth	Vaginal	W	No	No
Nancy	North Hospital	No	No	Emergency c-section, infant respiratory distress	Cesarean	W	No	No

(Continued)

Participant Name	Location of Birth	Transfer?	NICU Stay?	Other Complications	"Type" of Birth	Race*	Medicaid?**	Additional Children? (As of time of interview)
Renee	South Hospital	No	No	Two-vessel umbilical cord, unwanted c-section	Cesarean	W	No	No
Hannah	South Hospital	South Hospital to urban hospital (prior to birth)	Yes	Placental abruption, failed cervix	Cesarean	W	No	Three prior to BT (step-children)
Summer	South Hospital	No	No	Long labor, fetal distress, mastitis	Vaginal	W	No	No
Amber	South Hospital	No	No	Unwanted c-section, failed anesthesia	Cesarean	W	No	Multiple older adult children
Sue	North Hospital	North Hospital to urban (prior to birth)	Yes	Preterm, preeclampsia,	Vaginal	W	No	1 following BT
Kim	North Hospital	No	No	Stillbirth	Vaginal	W	No	Three prior to BT
Samantha	North Hospital	North Hospital to urban hospital (for infant)	Yes	Preterm birth, placental abruption, preeclampsia, emergency c-section	Cesarean	W	No	No
Natalie	Urban hospital	North Hospital to urban hospital	Yes	Emergency c-section, preterm birth, respiratory distress (infant)	Cesarean	W	No	No

(Continued)

Participant Name	Location of Birth	Transfer?	NICU Stay?	Other Complications	"Type" of Birth	Race*	Medicaid?**	Additional Children? (As of time of interview)
Kayla (two traumatic births)	First birth: Birth Center / Second birth: urban hospital	First birth: Birth center to North Hospital (for Mom) / Birth center to urban hospital (for infant)	Yes—both infants	First birth: infant respiratory distress, protruding uterus (Mom) / Second birth: IUGR infant, preterm birth, emergency c-section	Cesarean	W	No	No
Candace	South Hospital	No	No	Emergency c-section, preeclampsia	Cesarean	W	Yes	1 following BT
Joan	South Hospital	No	No	Gestational diabetes, fetal distress	Vacuum-assisted vaginal birth	W	No	2 prior to BT
Kathy	North Hospital	Home to hospital (prior to birth)	No	Hemorrhage, long labor	Vaginal	W	No	1 following BT
Phoebe	North Hospital	No	No	Long labor, fetal distress, forced suction	Vaginal — suction	W	Yes	1 prior to BT
Lori	North Hospital	Birth center to North Hospital (prior to birth)	No	Preeclampsia	Vaginal	W	No	No
Rhonda	North Hospital	No	No	Emergency c-section	Cesarean	W	No	1 following BT

(Continued)

Participant Name	Location of Birth	Transfer?	NICU Stay?	Other Complications	"Type" of Birth	Race*	Medicaid?**	Additional Children? (As of time of interview)
Melissa	North Hospital	No	No	Preeclampsia, emergency c-section	Cesarean	W	No	No
Trish	South Hospital	No	No	Emergency c-section, infant respiratory distress, mother hemorrhage	Cesarean	W	No	No
Tracy	South Hospital	No	No	Emergency c-section, long labor	Cesarean	W	No	2 prior to BT
Ashley	North Hospital	No	No	Preeclampsia, epidural failure, infant distress	Cesarean	W	No	No
Dee	North Hospital	North Hospital to urban hospital (prior to birth)	Yes	Preeclampsia, preterm birth	Vaginal	W	No	1 prior to BT, but first delivery (wife delivered first baby)
Jessica	Alaska	Transfer from local rural clinic to urban hospital	Yes	Preterm birth	Vaginal	W	Yes	1 prior to BT
Gail	Maryland	No	No	Emergency c-section, long labor	Cesarean	W	No	Two prior to traumatic birth

*We did not explicitly ask participants' race. Race here is based on perception from researchers.
**It is possible that additional participants were on Medicaid. We did not explicitly ask this question but those indicated self-disclosed that they used Medicaid.

Bibliography

42 CFR § 440.210. Required services for the categorically needy. https://www.law
.cornell.edu/cfr/text/42/440.210.

Abbassi-Ghanavati, Mina, James M. Alexander, Donald D. McIntire, Rashmin C.
Savani, and Kenneth J. Leveno. "Neonatal effects of magnesium sulfate given to
the mother." *American Journal of Perinatology* 29, no. 10 (2012): 795–800.

Affonso, Dyanne D., Anindya K. De, June Andrews Horowitz, and Linda J.
Mayberry. "An international study exploring levels of postpartum depressive
symptomatology." *Journal of Psychosomatic Research* 49, no. 3 (2000): 207–216.

Ahmed, Sara. *Complaint!* Durham, NC: Duke University Press, 2021.

Ahmed, Sara. "No" Accessed February 28, 2021, https://feministkilljoys.com/2017
/06/30/no/.

Ahmed, Sara. "Why Complain?" Feminist Killjoys. Accessed February 20, 2021 http:
//feministkilljoys.com/2019/07/22/why-complain.

Allen, Heidi, Bill J. Wright, Kristin Harding, and Lauren Broffman. "The role of
stigma in access to health care for the poor." *The Milbank Quarterly* 92, no. 2
(2014): 289–318.

Allers, Kimberley Seals. "Obstetric violence is a real problem. Evelyn Yang's experience is just one example." *The Washington Post.* February 6, 2020. Accessed
October 20, 2020. https://www.washingtonpost.com/lifestyle/2020/02/06/obstetric
-violence-is-real-problem-evelyn-yangs-experience-is-just-one-example/.

Always, Joan. "The Trouble with Gender: Tales of the Still-Missing Feminist
Revolution in Social Theory." *Sociological Theory* 13, no. 3 (1995): 209–228.

American College of Obstetricians and Gynecologists. "Ethical decision making
in obstetrics and gynecology." Committee Opinion No. 390, December 2007.
Accessed October 20, 2020. http://www.acog.org/from_home/ publications/ethics/
co390.pdf.

Anderson, Gerard F., Peter Hussey, and Varduhi Petrosyan. "It's still the prices,
stupid: why the US spends so much on health care, and a tribute to Uwe
Reinhardt." *Health Affairs* 38, no. 1 (2019): 87–95.

Anderson, Odin Waldemar. *The Uneasy Equilibrium: Private and Public Financing of Health Services in the United States, 1875-1965.* New College & Univ Pr, 1968.

Angel, Ronald, and Peter J. Guarnaccia. "Mind, body, and culture: Somatization among Hispanics." *Social Science & Medicine* 28, no. 12 (1989): 1229–1238.

Arendt, Hannah. *On Violence*, p. 36. New York: Harcourt, Brace, and Co., 1969.

Arendt, Hannah. *The Origins of Totalitarianism.* New York: Houghton Mifflin Harcourt Publishing Company, 1973.

Arendt, Hannah. *Eichmann in Jerusalem: A Report on the Banality of Evil.* New York: Penguin, 2006.

Arendt, Katherine, and Scott Segal. "Why epidurals do not always work." *Reviews in Obstetrics and Gynecology* 1, no. 2 (2008): 49.

Aron-Dine, Aviva. "New Research: Medicaid Expansion Saves Lives." Center on Budget and Policy Priorities. November 6, 2019. Accessed May 24th, 2020. https://www.cbpp.org/blog/new-research-medicaid-expansion-saves-lives.

Ayers, Susan. "Fear of childbirth, postnatal post-traumatic stress disorder and midwifery care." *Midwifery* 30, no. 2 (2014): 145–148.

Ayers, Susan, Andrew Eagle, and Helen Waring. "The effects of childbirth-related post-traumatic stress disorder on women and their relationships: a qualitative study." *Psychology, Health & Medicine* 11, no. 4 (2006): 389–398.

Ayers, Susan, Daniel B. Wright, and Nicola Wells. "Symptoms of post-traumatic stress disorder in couples after birth: association with the couple's relationship and parent–baby bond." *Journal of Reproductive and Infant Psychology* 25, no. 1 (2007): 40–50.

Baernholdt, Marianne, Bonnie Jennings, and Erica Lewis. "A Pilot Study of Staff Nurses' Perceptions of Factors that Influence Quality of Care in Critical Access Hospitals." *Journal of Nursing Care Quality* 28, no. 4 (2013): 352–359.

Beck, Cheryl. "Postpartum Depressed Mothers' Experiences Interacting with Their children." *Nursing Research* 45, no. 2 (1996): 98–104.

Beck, Cheryl Tatano, and Sue Watson. "Impact of birth trauma on breast-feeding: a tale of two pathways." *Nursing Research* 57, no. 4 (2008): 228–236.

Beckett, Katherine. "Choosing cesarean: Feminism and the politics of childbirth in the United States." *Feminist Theory* 6, no. 3 (2005): 251–275.

Bell, Aleeca F., and Ewa Andersson. "The birth experience and women's postnatal depression: a systematic review." *Midwifery* 39 (2016): 112–123.

Benatar, Solomon R. "Just healthcare beyond individualism: Challenges for North American bioethics." *Cambridge Q. Healthcare Ethics* 6 (1997): 397.

Bennett, Trude. "Reproductive health care in the rural United States." *Journal of the American Medical Association* 287, no. 1 (2002): 5.

Bernstein, Lenny. "How many patients should your doctor see each day." *The Washington Post.* May 22, 2014. Accessed November 20, 2020. https://www.washingtonpost.com/news/to-your-health/wp/2014/05/22/how-many-patients-should-your-doctor-see-each-day/.

Bernstein, Lenny. "U.S. faces 90,000 doctor shortage by 2025, medical school association warns." *The Washington Post.* March 3, 2015. Accessed July 8, 2020.

https://www.washingtonpost.com/news/to-your-health/wp/2015/03/03/u-s-faces-90000-doctor-shortage-by-2025-medical-school-association-warns/.

Beth Israel Lahey Health – Winchester Hospital. "Cystocele/Rectocele." Nd. Accessed October 19, 2020. https://www.winchesterhospital.org/health-library/article?id=100092.

Bordo, Susan. "Feminism, Foucault, and the politics of the body." In *Bodies and Pleasures*, edited by Ladelle McWhorter, 179–201. Bloomington, IN: Indiana University Press, 1999.

Bordo, Susan. *Unbearable Weight*. Berkley, CA: University of California Press, 2004.

Bucstain, Carmen, Gail Garmi, Noah Zafran, Sivan Zuarez-Easton, Julia Carmeli and Raed Salim. "Risk factors and perimpartum outcomes of failed epidural: A prospective cohort study." *Archives of Gynecology and Obstetrics* 295 (2017): 1119–1125.

Blumberg, Yoni. "Here's the real reason health care costs so much more in the U.S." *NBC*. Accessed Jun 18, 2020. https://www.cnbc.com/2018/03/22/the-real-reason-medical-care-costs-so-much-more-in-the-us.html.

Blumenthal, Susan. "The effects of socioeconomic status on health in rural and urban America." *Journal of the American Medical Association* 287, no. 1 (2002): 2.

Boucher, Debora, Catherine Bennett, Barbara McFarlin, and Rixa Freeze. "Staying home to give birth: why women in the United States choose home birth." *Journal of Midwifery & Women's Health* 54, no. 2 (2009): 119–126.

Bridges, Khiara. *Reproducing Race*. Berkeley: University of California Press, 2011.

Briggs, Laura. *Reproducing Empire: Race, Sex, Science, and US Imperialism in Puerto Rico*, vol. 11. Berkeley, CA: Univ of California Press, 2002.

Brockington, Ian. "Diagnosis and management of post-partum disorders: A review." *World Psychiatry* 3, no. 2 (2004): 89.

Brown, Brené. *Dare to Lead*. New York: Random House, 2018.

Butwick, Alexander J., Jason Bentley, Cynthia A. Wong, Jonathan M. Snowden, Eric Sun, and Nan Guo. "United States state-level variation in the use of neuraxial analgesia during labor for pregnant women." *JAMA Network Open* 1, no. 8 (2018): e186567–e186567.

Byatt, Nancy, Kathleen Biebel, Liz Friedman, Gifty Debordes-Jackson, and Douglas Ziedonis. "Women's perspectives on postpartum depression screening in pediatric settings: a preliminary study." *Archives of Women's Mental Health* 16, no. 5 (2013): 429–432.

Canton, Donald. *What a Blessing She Had Chloroform: The Medical and Social Response to the Pain of Childbirth from 1800 to the Present*. New Haven, CT: Yale University Press, 1999.

Carpentieri, Andrea M., James J. Lumalcuri, Jennie Shaw, and G. F. Joseph. "Overview of the 2015 American Congress of Obstetricians and Gynecologists' survey on professional liability." *Clin Rev* 20 (2015): 1–6.

Carroll, Aaron. "A doctor shortage? Let's take a closer look." *The New York Times*. November 7, 2016. Accessed July 9, 2020. https://www.nytimes.com/2016/11/08/upshot/a-doctor-shortage-lets-take-a-closer-look.html.

Center for Disease Control. "Births – Method of Delivery." Accessed September 3, 2020. https://www.cdc.gov/nchs/fastats/delivery.htm.

Center for Disease Control and Prevention. "Identifying Maternal Depression." Accessed November 21, 2020. https://www.cdc.gov/reproductivehealth/vital-signs/identifying-maternal-depression/index.html.

Center for Disease Control and Prevention. "Infant Mortality." March 27, 2019. https://www.cdc.gov/reproductivehealth/maternalinfanthealth/infantmortality.htm.

Center for Disease Control and Prevention. "Pregnancy Related Deaths." Accessed October 10, 2020. https://www.cdc.gov/reproductivehealth/maternalinfanthealth/pregnancy-relatedmortality.htm.

Center for Disease Control and Prevention. "Racial and Ethnic Disparities Continue in Pregnancy-Related Deaths." Accessed October 10, 2020. https://www.cdc.gov/media/releases/2019/p0905-racial-ethnic-disparities-pregnancy-deaths.html.

Center for Medicare and Medicaid Service. 2019. "Improving Access to Maternal Health Care in Rural Communities." Accessed November 5, 2020. https://www.cms.gov/About-CMS/Agency-Information/OMH/equity-initiatives/rural-health/09032019-Maternal-Health-Care-in-Rural-Communities.pdf.

Central Intelligence Agency. "Country Comparisons: Infant Mortality Rate" The World Factbook. Accessed November 8, 2020, https://www.cia.gov/library/Publications/the-world-factbook/fields/354rank.html.

Central Intelligence Agency. "Country Comparisons: Maternal Mortality Rate" The World Factbook. Accessed November 8, 2020. https://www.cia.gov/library/publications/the-world-factbook/rankorder/2223rank.html.

Cesarean Rates. "Understanding Cesarian Rates." Accessed September 25, 2020. https://www.cesareanrates.org.

Charles, Sonya. "Obstetricians and violence against women." *The American Journal of Bioethics* 11, no. 12 (2011): 51–56.

Chapman, Carleton B., and John M. Talmadge. "Historical and political background of federal health care legislation." *Law & Contemp. Probs.* 35 (1970): 334.

Chatterji, Pinka, and Sara Markowitz. *Family Leave after Childbirth and the Health of New Mothers*. No. w14156. National Bureau of Economic Research, 2008.

Cheng, Ching-Yu, Eileen R. Fowles, and Lorraine O. Walker. "Postpartum maternal health care in the United States: A critical review." *The Journal of Perinatal Education* 15, no. 3 (2006): 34.

Cixous, Hélène. "The Laugh of the Medusa." *Signs* 1, no. 4 (1976).

Coghlan, Andy. 2008. "C-sections may weaken bonding with baby." *The New Scientist*. September 4, 2008, https://www.newscientist.com/article/dn14662-c-sections-may-weaken-bonding-with-baby/.

Cogill, S. R., H. L. Caplan, Heather Alexandra, Kay Mordecai Robson, and R. Kumar. "Impact of maternal postnatal depression on cognitive development of young children." *British Medical Journal (Clin Res Ed)* 292, no. 6529 (1986): 1165–1167.

Cohn, Erika. 2020. "Belly of the Beast." In *APHA's 2020 VIRTUAL Annual Meeting and Expo* (Oct. 24–28). American Public Health Association, 2020.

Coldicott, Yvette, Britt-Ingjerd Nesheim, Jane MacDougall, Catherine Pope, and Clive Roberts. "The ethics of intimate examinations—teaching tomorrow's doctorsCommentary: Respecting the patient's integrity is the keyCommentary: Teaching pelvic examination—putting the patient first." *Bmj*326, no. 7380 (2003): 97–101.

Columbia Surgery. "History of Medicine: The Incubator Babies of Coney Island." *Columbia University.* Accessed July 6, 2020. https://columbiasurgery.org/news/20 15/08/06/history-medicine-incubator-babies-coney-island.

Commissioned Corps of the U.S. Public Health Service. "Our History." Accessed November 17, 2020. https://www.usphs.gov/aboutus/history.aspx.

Cook, Katie and Loomis, Collen. "The impact of choice and control on women's childbirth experiences." *Journal of Parinatal Education* 21, no. 3 (2012): 158–168.

Cosgrove, Lisa, and Akansha Vaswani. "Fetal rights, the policing of pregnancy, and meanings of the maternal in an age of neoliberalism." *Journal of Theoretical and Philosophical Psychology* 40, no. 1 (2020): 43.

Creedy, Debra K., Ian M. Shochet, and Jan Horsfall. "Childbirth and the development of acute trauma symptoms: incidence and contributing factors." *Birth* 27, no. 2 (2000): 104–111.

Côté-Arsenault, Denise and Marsha Mason Freije. "Support groups help women through pregnancies after loss." *Western Journal of Nursing Research* 26, no. 6 (2004), DOI: 10.1177/0193945904265817.

Czarnocka, Jo, and Pauline Slade. "Prevalence and predictors of post-traumatic stress symptoms following childbirth." *British Journal of Clinical Psychology* 39, no. 1 (2000): 35–51.

D'Emilio, J. 1983. *Sexual Politics, Sexual Communities.* Chicago, IL: University of Chicago Press.

Davies, John, Pauline Slade, Ingram Wright, and Peter Stewart. "Posttraumatic stress symptoms following childbirth and mothers' perceptions of their infants." *Infant Mental Health Journal: Official Publication of The World Association for Infant Mental Health* 29, no. 6 (2008): 537–554.

Davis, Karen; Kristof Stremikis, David Squires, and Cathy Schoen. "Mirror, Mirror on the Wall." *The Commonwealth Fund.* June 2014. Accessed June 6, 2020. https://www.commonwealthfund.org/sites/default/files/documents/___media_files _publications_fund_report_2014_jun_1755_davis_mirror_mirror_2014.pdf.

Dawson, Drew, and Kathryn Reid. "Fatigue, alcohol and performance impairment." *Nature* 388, no. 6639 (1997): 235–235.

De Carvalho Guerra Abecasis, Francisco, and Antonio Gomes. "Rooming-in for preterm infants: How far should we go? Five-year experience at a tertiary hospital." *Acta Paediatrica* 95, no. 12 (2006): 1567–1570.

De Vries, Raymond, Cecilia Benoit, Edwin Van Teijlingen, and Sirpa Wrede, eds. *Birth by Design: Pregnancy, Maternity Care and Midwifery in North America and Europe.* Routledge, 2002.

Declercq, Eugene R., Carol Sakala, Maureen P. Corry, S. Applebaum, and Peter Risher. "Listening to mothers: Report of the first national US survey of women's childbearing experiences." *New York* (2002).

DeKeseredy, Walter S., Stephen L. Muzzatti, and Joseph F. Donnermeyer. "Mad men in bib overalls: Media's horrification and pornification of rural culture." *Critical Criminology* 22, no. 2 (2014): 179–197.

Delker, Brianna C., Rowan Salton, and Kate C. McLean. "Giving voice to silence: Empowerment and disempowerment in the developmental shift from trauma 'victim' to 'survivor-advocate.'" *Journal of Trauma & Dissociation* 21, no. 2 (2020): 242–263.

Denis, Anne, Olivier Parant, and Stacey Callahan. "Post-traumatic stress disorder related to birth: a prospective longitudinal study in a French population." *Journal of Reproductive and Infant Psychology* 29, no. 2 (2011): 125–135.

Diaz-Tello, Farah. "Invisible wounds: obstetric violence in the United States." *Reproductive health matters* 24, no. 47 (2016): 56–64.

Dis, Jane van. "Editors Note." *Journal of the American Medical Association* 287, no. 1 (2002): 1.

Donegan, Jane B. "'Safe Delivered,' but by Whom? Midwives and Men-midwives in Early America." In *Women and Health in America: Historical Readings*, edited by Judith Walzer Leavitt, 302–317. Madison, WI: University of Wisconsin Press, 1984.

Dye, Nancy Schrom. "History of Childbirth in America." *Signs* 6, no. 1 (1980): 97–108.

Eberhardt, Mark Stephen, Virginia M. Freid, Sam Harper, Deborah D. Ingram, Diane M. Makuc, Elsie Pamuk, and Kate Prager. "Health, United States, 2001, with urban and rural health chartbook." (2001).

Escobar, Javier I., Glorisa Canino, Maritza Rubio-Stipec, and Milagros Bravo. "Somatic symptoms after a natural disaster: A prospective study." *The American Journal of Psychiatry* (1992).

Edwards, Denzil RL, Sally-Anne M. Porter, and George S. Stein. "A pilot study of postnatal depression following caesarean section using two retrospective self-rating instruments." *Journal of psychosomatic research* 38, no. 2 (1994): 111–117.

Elmir, Rakime, Virginia Schmied, Lesley Wilkes, and Debra Jackson. "Women's perceptions and experiences of a traumatic birth: A meta-ethnography." *Journal of Advanced Nursing* 66, no. 10 (2010): 2142–2153.

Essex, Marilyn J., Marjorie H. Klein, Eunsuk Cho, and Ned H. Kalin. "Maternal stress beginning in infancy may sensitize children to later stress exposure: Effects on cortisol and behavior." *Biological psychiatry* 52, no. 8 (2002): 776–784.

Evins, G. G., Theofrastous, J. P., & Galvin, S. L. "Postpartum depression: A comparison of screening and routine clinical evaluation." *American Journal of Obstetrics and Gynecology* 182, no. 5 (2000): 1080–1082.

Feeley, Nancy, Phyllis Zelkowitz, Carole Cormier, Lyne Charbonneau, Annie Lacroix, and Apostolos Papageorgiou. "Posttraumatic stress among mothers of very low birthweight infants at 6 months after discharge from the neonatal intensive care unit." *Applied Nursing Research* 24, no. 2 (2011): 114–117.

Fielding, Sarah. "What America can learn from the mental health care systems of other countries." *Talk Space.* April 6, 2020. Accessed November 8, 2020. https://www.talkspace.com/blog/america-mental-health-care-systems/.

Finish Medical Association. "Overview of the healthcare system in Finland." *Health Management* 7, no. 5 (2007). https://healthmanagement.org/c/imaging/issuearticle/overview-of-the-healthcare-system-in-finland.

Flinn, Fiona, and Claire Armstrong. "Junior doctors' extended work hours and the effects on their performance: The Irish case." *International Journal for Quality in Health Care* 23, no. 2 (2011): 210–217.

Fisher, Lawrence. "Developing health care within the context of primary care." *Archives of Family Medicine* 6 (1997): 324–333.

Forcada-Guex, Margarita, Ayala Borghini, Blaise Pierrehumbert, François Ansermet, and Carole Muller-Nix. "Prematurity, maternal posttraumatic stress and consequences on the mother–infant relationship." *Early Human Development* 87, no. 1 (2011): 21–26.

Foucault, Michel. *Discipline and Punish.* New York: Random House, 1977.

Foucault, Michel. *Discipline and Punish: The Birth of the Prison.* New York: Penguin, 1991.

Foucault, Michel. *The History of Sexuality*, vol. 1. New York: Vintage, 1998.

Foucault, Michel. *Society Must be Defended: Lectures at the College de France 1975-1976.* New York: Picador Press, 2003.

Foucault, Michel. *The Essential Foucault: Selections from Essential Works of Foucault, 19540 1984.* New York: The New Press, 2003.

Fox, Bonnie, and Diana Worts. "Revisiting the critique of medicalized childbirth: A contribution to the sociology of birth." *Gender & Society* 13, no. 3 (1999): 326–346.

Fuller, Cheryl A., and Robin Gallagher. "What's happening: Perceived benefits and barriers of prenatal care in low income women." *Journal of the American Association of Nurse Practitioners* 11, no. 12 (1999): 527.

Garthus-Niegel, Susan, Susan Ayers, Julia Martini, Tilmann von Soest, and Malin Eberhard-Gran. "The impact of postpartum post-traumatic stress disorder symptoms on child development: a population-based, 2-year follow-up study." *Psychological Medicine* 47 (2017): 161–170.

Glaser, Barney and Anselm Strauss. *The Discovery of Grounded Theory.* New York: Routledge, 2017.

Goodyear, Sheena. "This former U.S. health insurance exec says he lied to Americans about Canadian health care." *As it Happens, Canadian Broadcast Corporation.* June 29, 2020. Accessed November 22, 2020 https://www.cbc.ca/radio/asithappens/as-it-happens-monday-edition-1.5631285/this-former-u-s-health-insurance-exec-says-he-lied-to-americans-about-canadian-health-care-1.5631874.

Gottlieb, Joshua D., Adam Hale Shapiro, and Abe Dunn. "The complexity of billing and paying for physician care." *Health Affairs* 37, no. 4 (2018): 619–626.

Gottvall, Karin, and Ulla Waldenström. "Does a traumatic birth experience have an impact on future reproduction?." *BJOG: An International Journal of Obstetrics and Gynaecology* 109, no. 3 (2002): 254–260.

Gramsci, Antonio. *The Prison Notebooks.* London: Lawrence and Wishard, 1971.

Guardado, José. "Medical liability claims frequency among U.S. physicians." *American Medical Association.* Accessed November 21, 2020. https://www.ama-assn.org/practice-management/sustainability/medical-liability-market-research.

Guerriero, Wm. "Early Controlled Ambulation in the Puerperium." *American Journal of Obstetrics and Gynecology* 51 (1948): 312–313.

Guinier, Lani and Gerald Torres. *The Miner's Canary: Enlisting Race, Resisting Power, Transforming Democracy*, 252. Harvard University Press, 2009.

Gulamani, Salima S., Shahirose Sadrudin Premji, ZeenatKhanu Kanji, and Syed Iqbal Azam. "A review of postpartum depression, preterm birth, and culture." *The Journal of Perinatal & Neonatal Nursing* 27, no. 1 (2013): 52–59.

Harris, Rachel, and Susan Ayers. "What makes labour and birth traumatic? A survey of intrapartum 'hotspots.'" *Psychology & Health* 27, no. 10 (2012): 1166–1177.

Harrison, Wade, and David Goodman. "Epidemiologic trends in neonatal intensive care, 2007-2012." *JAMA Pediatrics* 169, no. 9 (2015): 855–862.

He, Xiaojia, Luma Akil, Winfred G. Aker, Huey-Min Hwang, and Hafiz A. Ahmad. "Trends in infant mortality in United States: A brief study of the southeastern states from 2005–2009." *International Journal of Environmental Research and Public Health* 12, no. 5 (2015): 4908–4920.

Heady, Hilda R. "A delicate balance: The economics of rural health care delivery." *JAMA* 287, no. 1 (2002): 110–110.

Health Direct. "Treating pre-eclampsia." Accessed June 8, 2020. https://www.pregnancybirthbaby.org.au/treating-pre-eclampsia.

Heiser, Stuart. "New Findings Confirm Predictions on Physician Shortage." *AAMC*. April 23, 2019. Accessed June 7, 2020. https://www.aamc.org/news-insights/press-releases/new-findings-confirm-predictions-physician-shortage.

Heller, Kevin Jon. "Power, subjectification and resistance in Foucault." *SubStance* 25, no. 1 (1996): 78–110.

Himmelstein, David U., Robert M. Lawless, Deborah Thorne, Pamela Foohey, and Steffie Woolhandler. "Medical bankruptcy: still common despite the Affordable Care Act." (2019): 431–433.

Hoadley, Jack, Joan Alker, and Mark Holmes. "Health insurance coverage in small towns and rural America." Georgetown University Center for Children and Families and the University of North Carolina. NC Rural Health Research Program. Accessed September 9, 2020. https://ccf.georgetown.edu/wp-content/uploads/2018/09/FINALHealthInsuranceCoverage_Rural_2018.pdf.

Hoang, Giao N., and Roy V. Erickson. "Guidelines for providing medical care to Southeast Asian refugees." *Jama*248, no. 6 (1982): 710–714.

Hoge, Elizabeth A., Sharad M. Tamrakar, Kelly M. Christian, Namrata Mahara, Mahendra K. Nepal, Mark H. Pollack, and Naomi M. Simon. "Cross-cultural differences in somatic presentation in patients with generalized anxiety disorder." *The Journal of Nervous and Mental Disease* 194, no. 12 (2006): 962–966.

Holdren, Sarah, Cynthia Fair, and Liisa Lehtonen. "A qualitative cross-cultural analysis of NICU care culture and infant feeding in Finland and the US." *BMC Pregnancy and Childbirth* 19, no. 1 (2019): 1–12.

Holtz, Bree, Andrew Smock and David Reyes-Gastelum. "Connected motherhood: Social support for moms and moms-to-be on Facebook." *Telemedicine and e-Health* 21, no. 5 (2015), https://www.liebertpub.com/doi/abs/10.1089/tmj.2014.0118.

Horlocker, Terese T., Martin D. Abel, Joseph M. Messick Jr, and Darrell R. Schroeder. "Small risk of serious neurologic complications related to lumbar epidural catheter placement in anesthetized patients." *Anesthesia & Analgesia* 96, no. 6 (2003): 1547–1552.

Horwitz, Allan V. "The sociological study of mental illness." In *Handbook of the Sociology of Mental Health*, edited by C. Aneshensel, J. Phelan, and A. Bierman, 57–78. Boston, MA: Springer, 1999.

Howard, Jacqueline. "C-section deliveries nearly doubled worldwide since 2000, study finds." *CNN.* October 11, 2018. https://www.cnn.com/2018/10/11/health/c-section-rates-study-parenting-without-borders-intl/index.html.

Hsu, Elizabeth. "Medical Pluralism." In *International Encyclopedia of Public Health.* 2nd Edition, edited by Stella Quah, 8–12. Academic Press, 2016.

Institute for Quality and Efficiency in Health Care. "Pregnancy and birth: Epidurals and painkillers for labor pain relief." March 22, 2018. Available from: https://www.ncbi.nlm.nih.gov/books/NBK279567/.

Institute of Medicine. *Employment and Health Benefits: A Connection at Risk.* Washington, DC: The National Academies Press, 1993.

Institute of Medicine (US) Committee on the Consequences of Uninsurance. *Care Without Coverage: Too Little, Too Late.* Washington, DC: National Academies Press, 2002.

Ionio, Chiara, and Paola Di Blasio. "Post-traumatic stress symptoms after childbirth and early mother–child interactions: An exploratory study." *Journal of Reproductive and Infant Psychology* 32, no. 2 (2014): 163–181.

Jacobson, Roni. "Widespread understaffing of nurses increases risk to patients." *Scientific American* July 14, 2015.

Jindia, Shilpa. "Belly of the Beast: California's dark history of forced sterilizations." *The Guardian.* June 30, 2020. Accessed October 1, 2020. https://www.theguardian.com/us-news/2020/jun/30/california-prisons-forced-sterilizations-belly-beast.

Jorgensen, Anne. "Born in the USA – The History of Neonatology in the United States: A Century of Caring." *NICU Currents.* 2010. Accessed June 20, 2020. https://static.abbottnutrition.com/cms-prod/anhi-2017.org/img/history-of-neonatology_tcm1423-102720.pdf.

Kafka, Franz. 2011. *The Trial.* New York: Tribeca Books, 2011.

Kane, Pratibha P. "Stress causing psychosomatic illness among nurses." *Indian Journal of Occupational and Environmental Medicine* 13, no. 1 (2009): 28.

Katz, Michael. *The Undeserving Poor.* Oxford: Oxford University Press, 2013.

Kemppainen, Laura, Teemu Kemppainen, Natalia Skogberg, Hannamaria Kuusio, and Päivikki Koponen. "Immigrants', use of health care in their country of origin: the role of social integration, discrimination and the parallel use of health care systems." *Scandinavian Journal of Caring Sciences* 32, no. 2 (2018): 698–706.

Kessler, Ronald C., Olga Demler, Richard G. Frank, Mark Olfson, Harold Alan Pincus, Ellen E. Walters, Philip Wang, Kenneth B. Wells, and Alan M. Zaslavsky. "Prevalence and treatment of mental disorders, 1990 to 2003." *New England Journal of Medicine* 352, no. 24 (2005): 2515–2523.

Kiser, Laurel J., Barbara Baumgardner, and Joyce Dorado. "Who are we, but for the stories we tell: Family stories and healing." *Psychological Trauma: Theory, Research, Practice, and Policy* 2, no. 3 (2010): 243.

Ko, Lisa. "Unwanted sterilization and eugenics programs in the United States." *Independent Lens.* January 29, 2016. Accessed October 10, 2020. https://www.pbs.org/independentlens/blog/unwanted-sterilization-and-eugenics-programs-in-the-united-states/.

Konish, Lorie. 2019. "This is the real reason most Americans file for bankruptcy." CNBC. February 11, 2019. Accessed May 24, 2020. https://www.cnbc.com/2019/02/11/this-is-the-real-reason-most-americans-file-for-bankruptcy.html.

Korja, Riikka, Elina Savonlahti, Sari Ahlqvist-Björkroth, Suvi Stolt, Leena Haataja, Helena Lapinleimu, Jorma Piha, Liisa Lehtonen, and PIPARI Study Group. "Maternal depression is associated with mother–infant interaction in preterm infants." *Acta Paediatrica* 97, no. 6 (2008): 724–730.

Kotaska, Andrew. "Informed consent and refusal in obstetrics: A practical ethical guide." *Birth* 44, no. 3 (2017): 195–199.

Kozhimannil, Katy Backes, Julia D. Interrante, Carrie Henning-Smith, and Lindsay K. Admon. "Rural-urban differences in severe maternal morbidity and mortality in the US, 2007–15." *Health Affairs* 38, no. 12 (2019): 2077–2085.

Kringos, Dionne S., Wienke GW Boerma, Allen Hutchinson, and Richard B. Saltman. *Building Primary Care in a Changing Europe. Case studies.* WHO Regional Office for Europe, 2015.

Kukura, Elizabeth. "Obstetric violence." *Georgetown Law Journal* 106 (2017): 721.

Kuznia, Robert, Nelli Black, and Drew Griffin. "Evelyn Yang says Columbia University and New York DA 'grossly mishandled' case of OB-GYN she accuses of sexual assault." *CNN.* February 21, 2020. Accessed October 18, 2020. https://www.cnn.com/2020/02/21/politics/evelyn-yang-marissa-hoechstetter-vance-invs/index.html.

Lamaze International. "What is Obstetric Violence and What if it Happens to you?" July 20, 2020. Accessed October 19, 2020. https://www.lamaze.org/Giving-Birth-with-Confidence/GBWC-Post/what-is-obstetric-violence-and-what-if-it-happens-to-you.

Leavitt, Judith. "'Science' Enters the Birthing Room." *The Journal of American History* 70, no. 2 (1983): 281–304.

Leavitt, Judith Walzer. "Birthing and anesthesia: The debate over twilight sleep," *Signs* 6, no. 1 (1984): 147–164.

Lee, Helena. "Why Finnish babies sleep in cardboard boxes." *BBC News* June 4, 2013. Accessed November 1, 2020. https://www.bbc.com/news/magazine-22751415.

Lerman, Sheera F., Golan Shahar, Kathryn A. Czarkowski, Naamit Kurshan, Urania Magriples, Linda C. Mayes, and C. Neill Epperson. "Predictors of satisfaction with obstetric care in high-risk pregnancy: The importance of patient–provider relationship." *Journal of Clinical Psychology in Medical Settings* 14, no. 4 (2007): 330–334.

Lester, Felicia. "Why is Maternal Mortality so High in the U.S.?" University of California – Berkeley. Accessed June 6, 2020. https://www.berkeleywellness.com/healthy-community/health-care-policy/article/why-maternal-mortality-so-high-us.

Levine, David. 2018. "How much of a struggle is it to get mental health care in rural areas?" *U.S. News and World Report.* April 20. Accessed November 5, 2020. https ://health.usnews.com/health-care/patient-advice/articles/2018-04-20/how-much -of-a-struggle-is-it-to-get-mental-health-care-in-rural-areas.

Levy, Gabrielle. "Dying to be Heard." *US News and World Report.* April 20, 2018. https://www.usnews.com/news/the-report/articles/2018-04-20/why-women-strugg le-to-get-doctors-to-believe-them.

Lim, Stephen S., Rachel L. Updike, Alexander S. Kaldjian, Ryan M. Barber, Krycia Cowling, Hunter York, Joseph Friedman et al. "Measuring human capital: A systematic analysis of 195 countries and territories, 1990–2016." *The Lancet* 392, no. 10154 (2018): 1217–1234.

Lin, E. H., William B. Carter, and Arthur M. Kleinman. "An exploration of somatization among Asian refugees and immigrants in primary care." *American Journal of Public Health* 75, no. 9 (1985): 1080–1084.

Livingston, Gretchen and Thomas, Deja. "Among 41 countries, only U.S. lacks paid parental leave." Pew Research Center. December 16, 2019. Accessed November 5, 2020. https://www.pewresearch.org/fact-tank/2019/12/16/u-s-lacks-mandated-paid -parental-leave/.

Lockley, Steven W., Laura K. Barger, Najib T. Ayas, Jeffrey M. Rothschild, Charles A. Czeisler, and Christopher P. Landrigan. "Effects of health care provider work hours and sleep deprivation on safety and performance." *The Joint Commission Journal on Quality and Patient Safety* 33, no. 11 (2007): 7–18.

Lukas, Martin. "Neoliberalism has conned us into fighting climate change as individuals." *The Guardian.* July 17, 2017. https://www.theguardian.com/environ ment/true-north/2017/jul/17/neoliberalism-has-conned-us-into-fighting-climate-ch ange-as-individuals.

Luker, Sarah. *Salsa Dancing in the Social Sciences: Research in an Age of Info-Glut.* Cambridge, MA: Harvard University Press, 2008.

MacDorman, Marian F, and Eugene Declercq. "Trends and state variations in out-of-hospital births in the United States, 2004-2017." *Birth* 46 no. 2 (2019): 279–288.

MacDorman, Marian F., T. J. Mathews, Ashna D. Mohangoo, and Jennifer Zeitlin. "International comparisons of infant mortality and related factors: United States and Europe, 2010." (2014).

Macdougall, Christiana. "'Oh, Get Over It. I Do This Every Day': How Ignoring the Specialness of Childbirth Contributes to Experiences of Emotional Distress." *Journal of the Motherhood Initiative for Research and Community Involvement* 9, no. 2 (2018).

Mahadeo, Rahsaan. "Funk the Clock: Transgressing Time While Young, Prescient and Black." University of Minnesota Dissertations (2019).

Makary, Marty. *The Price We Pay: What Broke American Health Care – and How.* New York: Bloomsbury, 2019.

Malin, Maili, and Mika Gissler. "Maternal care and birth outcomes among ethnic minority women in Finland." *BMC Public Health* 9, no. 1 (2009), DOI: 10.1186/1471-2458-9-84.

March of Dimes. "Prenatal Tests." Accessed June 5, 2020. https://www.marchofd
imes.org/pregnancy/prenatal-tests.aspx.

Martell, Louise. "The Hospital and the Postpartum Experience: A Historical Analysis." *Journal of Obstetric, Gynecologic, and Neonatal Nursing* 29, no. 1 (2000): 65–72.

Martell, Louise. "Maternity Care During the Post World War II Baby Boom," 387–404.

Martin, Joyce A., Brady E. Hamilton, Michelle JK Osterman, Sally C. Curtin, and T. J. Mathews. "Births: Final data for 2013 (National Vital Statistics Reports, Vol. 64, No. 1)." *Hyattsville, MD: National Center for Health Statistics* (2015).

Martins, Carla and Elizabeth A. Gaffan. "Effects of early maternal depression on patterns of infant-mother attachment: A meta-analytic investigation." *Journal of Child Psychology and Psychiatry* 41, no. 6 (2000): 737–746.

Mattingly, Susan S. "The maternal-fetal dyad exploring the two-patient obstetric model." *The Hastings Center Report* 22, no. 1 (1992): 13–18. Accessed October 16, 2020. DOI:10.2307/3562716.

Maxwell, December, Sarah R. Robinson, and Kelli Rogers. "'I keep it to myself': A qualitative meta-interpretive synthesis of experiences of postpartum depression among marginalised women." *Health & Social Care in the Community* 27, no. 3 (2019): e23–e36.

Mayer, Caroline. "The Health Claim Game." *AARP Magazine.* Nov/Dec 2009. https://www.aarp.org/health/medicare-insurance/info-09-2009/health_claim_game.html.

Mazzula, Silvia L., and Rebecca R. Campón. "Microaggressions: Toxic Rain in Health Care." *Microaggression Theory: Influence and Implications* (2018): 108.

McIntosh, James. "Models of childbirth and social class: A study of 80 working-class primigravidae." In *Midwives, Research and Childbirth*, edited by S. Robinson and A. Thomson, 189–214. Boston, MA: Springer, 1989.

Medscape. "Medscape physician compensation report 2019." Accessed July 7, 2020. https://www.medscape.com/slideshow/2019-compensation-ob-gyn-6011337#17.

Meserve, Emily E., Mana M. Parast, and Theonia K. Boyd. "Gestational diseases and the placenta." In *Diagnostic Gynecologic and Obstetric Pathology*, 1219–1249. Content Repository Only, 2018.

Miller, Amy Chasteen, and Thomas E. Shriver. "Women's childbirth preferences and practices in the United States." *Social Science & Medicine* 75, no. 4 (2012): 709–716.

Mirkovic, Kelsey R., Cria G. Perrine, Kelley S. Scanlon, and Laurence M. Grummer-Strawn. "Maternity leave duration and full-time/part-time work status are associated with US mothers' ability to meet breastfeeding intentions." *Journal of Human Lactation* 30, no. 4 (2014): 416–419.

Molina, George, Thomas G. Weiser, Stuart R. Lipsitz, Micaela M. Esquivel, Tarsicio Uribe-Leitz, Tej Azad, Neel Shah et al. "Relationship between cesarean delivery rate and maternal and neonatal mortality." *Jama* 314, no. 21 (2015): 2263–2270.

Mollica, Richard R. "The trauma story: The psychiatric care of refugee survivors of violence and torture." In *Post-Traumatic Therapy and Victims of Violence*, edited by F. Ochberg, 295–314. New York: Brunner/Mazel, 1988.

Mozurkewich, Ellen. "Working conditions and pregnancy outcomes: An updated appraisal of the evidence." *American Journal of Obstetrics & Gynecology* 222, no. 3 (2020): 201–203.

Muller-Nix, Carole, Margarita Forcada-Guex, Blaise Pierrehumbert, Lyne Jaunin, Ayala Borghini, and François Ansermet. "Prematurity, maternal stress and mother–child interactions." *Early Human Development* 79, no. 2 (2004): 145–158.

Murray, Lynne, Peter Cooper, and Alison Hipwell. "Mental health of parents caring for infants." *Archives of Women's Mental Health* 6, no. 2 (2003): s71–s77.

N.A. "Celebrity C-sections: Guess who's too posh to push." *Orlando Sentinel.* N.d. Accessed November 20, 2020. https://www.orlandosentinel.com/features/family/orl-celebrities-csections-moms-photos-photogallery.html.

National Academies of Sciences, Engineering, and Medicine; Health and Medicine Division; Division of Behavioral and Social Sciences and Education; Board on Children, Youth, and Families; Committee on Assessing Health Outcomes by Birth Settings; Backes EP, Scrimshaw SC, editors. *Birth Settings in America: Outcomes, Quality, Access, and Choice.* Washington, DC: National Academies Press, 2020.

National Advisory Committee on Rural Health and Human Services. "Maternal and Obstetric care challenges in rural America." Accessed November 5, 2020. https://www.hrsa.gov/sites/default/files/hrsa/advisory-committees/rural/publicat ions/2020-maternal-obstetric-care-challenges.pdf.

National Rural Health Association. "About Rural Health Care." Accessed August 20, 2020. https://www.ruralhealthweb.org/about-nrha/about-rural-health-care.

Nelson, Margaret K. "Working-class women, middle-class women, and models of childbirth." *Social Problems* 30, no. 3 (1983): 284–297.

Nicholls, Karen, and Susan Ayers. "Childbirth-related post-traumatic stress disorder in couples: A qualitative study." *British Journal of Health Psychology* 12, no. 4 (2007): 491–509.

Nilsson, Christina, Eva Robertson, and Ingela Lundgren. "An Effort to Make All the Pieces Come Together: Women's Long-Term Perspectives on Their Experiences of Intense Fear of Childbirth." *International Journal of Childbirth* 2, no. 4 (2012): 255–268.

O'Cathain Alicia, Thomas Kate, Walters Stephen, Nicholl Jon, and Kirkham Mavis. "Women's perceptions of informed choice in maternity care." *Midwifery* 18, no. 2 (2002): 136–144.

OECD/European Observatory on Health Systems and Policies. 2017. "State of the Health of the EU: Finland." OECD Publishing. Paris/European Observatory on Health Systems and Policies, Brussels. http://dx.doi.org/10.1787/978926428 3367-en.

Office of the Surgeon General (US); Center for Mental Health Services (US); National Institute of Mental Health (US). "Chapter 2 Culture Counts: The Influence of Culture and Society on Mental Health." *Mental Health: Culture, Race, and Ethnicity: A Supplement to Mental Health: A Report of the Surgeon General.* Rockville, MD: Substance Abuse and Mental Health Services Administration, 2001. Available from: https://www.ncbi.nlm.nih.gov/books/NBK44249/.

Olde, Eelco, Onno van der Hart, Rolf Kleber, and Maarten van Son. "Posttraumatic stress following childbirth: A review." *Clinical Psychology Review* 26, no. 1 (2006): 1–16.

Ospina, Naykky Singh, Kari A. Phillips, Rene Rodriguez-Gutierrez, Ana Castaneda-Guarderas, Michael R. Gionfriddo, Megan E. Branda, and Victor M. Montori. "Eliciting the patient's agenda-secondary analysis of recorded clinical encounters." *Journal of General Internal Medicine* 34, no. 1 (2019): 36–40.

Osterman, Michelle JK, and Joyce A. Martin. "Trends in low-risk cesarean delivery in the United States, 1990-2013." (2014).

Ollove, Michael. "A shortage in the Nation's Maternal Health Care." The Pew Charitable Trust. August 15, 2016. Accessed July 10, 2020. https://www.pewtrusts .org/en/research-and-analysis/blogs/stateline/2016/08/15/a-shortage-in-the-nations -maternal-health-care.

Ollove, Michael. "A Showing number of U.S. women still die of childbirth. California is doing something about that." *Washington Post.* November 4, 2018. https:// www.washingtonpost.com/national/health-science/a-shocking-number-of-us-w omen-still-die-from-childbirth-california-is-doing-something-about-that/2018/11/ 02/11042036-d7af-11e8-a10f-b51546b10756_story.html.

Organization for Economic Co-operation and Development. "Health Spending." Accessed June 20, 2020. https://data.oecd.org/healthres/health-spending.htm.

Pagán, Camille. "When Doctors Downplay Women's Health Concerns." *New York Times.* May 3, 2018. https://www.nytimes.com/2018/05/03/well/live/when-doctors -downplay-womens-health-concerns.html.

Panagioti, Maria, Keith Geraghty, Judith Johnson, Anli Zhou, Efharis Panagopoulou, Carolyn Chew-Graham, David Peters, Alexander Hodkinson, Ruth Riley, and Aneez Esmail. "Association between physician burnout and patient safety, professionalism, and patient satisfaction: a systematic review and meta-analysis." *JAMA internal medicine* 178, no. 10 (2018): 1317–1331.

Paul, Ian M., Danielle S. Downs, Eric W. Schaefer, Jessica S. Beiler, and Carol S. Weisman. "Postpartum anxiety and maternal-infant health outcomes." *Pediatrics* 131, no. 4 (2013): e1218–e1224.

Parfitt, Ylva, Susan Ayers, Alison Pike, D. C. Jessop, and Elizabeth Ford. "A prospective study of the parent–baby bond in men and women 15 months after birth." *Journal of Reproductive and Infant Psychology* 32, no. 5 (2014): 441–456.

Park, Ryan. "Why so many young doctors work such awful hours." *The Atlantic.* February 21, 2017. Accessed July 6, 2020. https://www.theatlantic.com/business/ archive/2017/02/doctors-long-hours-schedules/516639/.

Patel, Rikinkumar S., Ramya Bachu, Archana Adikey, Meryem Malik, and Mansi Shah. "Factors related to physician burnout and its consequences: A review." *Behavioral Sciences* 8, no. 11 (2018): 98.

Pattani, Aneri. "Silenced by Fear." *The Philadelphia Inquirer.* April 5 2019. https://www.inquirer.com/health/a/postpartum-depression-perinatal-mental-he alth-new-mom-women-of-color-20190405.html.

Paul, Tanya A. "Prevalence of posttraumatic stress symptoms after childbirth: does ethnicity have an impact?." *The Journal of perinatal education* 17, no. 3 (2008): 17–26. DOI:10.1624/105812408X324534.

Pearlstein, Teri, Margaret Howard, Amy Salisbury, and Caron Zlotnick. "Postpartum depression." *American Journal of Obstetrics and Gynecology* 200, no. 4 (2009): 357–364.

Pilgeram, Ryanne. *Pushed Out: Contested Development and Rural Gentrification in the US West.* Seattle, WA: University of Washington Press, 2021.

Polletta, Francesca, and James M. Jasper. "Collective identity and social movements." *Annual Review of Sociology* 27, no. 1 (2001): 283–305.

Preskey, Natasha. "Why are women still refusing painkillers during childbirth? *Vice.* January 3, 2019. Accessed November 21, 2020. https://www.vice.com/en_us/art icle/439mvm/this-is-why-the-natural-birth-movement-isnt-slowing-down.

Primary Care Collaborative. 2020. "Benefits of Integration of Behavioral Health." Accessed November 8, 2020. https://www.pcpcc.org/content/benefits-integration -behavioral-health.

Public Broadcasting System. "Health Care Crisis: Who's at Risk?" Accessed November 20, 2020. https://www.pbs.org/healthcarecrisis/.

Pyykönen, Aura, Mika Gissler, Ellen Løkkegaard, Thomas Bergholt, Steen C. Rasmussen, Alexander Smárason, Ragnheiður I. Bjarnadóttir et al. "Cesarean section trends in the Nordic Countries–a comparative analysis with the Robson classification." *Acta obstetricia et gynecologica Scandinavica* 96, no. 5 (2017): 607–616.

Rabinowitz, Howard and Paynter, Nina. "Reproductive health care in the rural United States." *Journal of the American Medical Association* 287, no. 1 (2002): 6.

Radu, Sintia. "Countries with the most well-developed health care systems." *U.S. News and World Report.* January 21, 2020. Accessed July 6, 2020. https://ww w.usnews.com/news/best-countries/slideshows/countries-with-the-most-well-de veloped-public-health-care-system?onepage.

Ragan, Charles. *The Comparative Method: moving Beyond Qualitative and Quantitative Strategies.* Berkeley, CA: University of California Press, 1987.

Rai, Shashi, Abhishek Pathak, and Indira Sharma. "Postpartum psychiatric disorders: Early diagnosis and management." *Indian Journal of Psychiatry* 57, no. Suppl 2 (2015): S216.

Redden, Molly. "New York hospital's secret policy led to woman being given c-section against her will." *The Guardian.* October 5, 2017. Accessed September 30, 2020. https://www.theguardian.com/us-news/2017/oct/05/new-york-staten-island -university-hospital-c-section-ethics-medicine; https://www.glamour.com/story/ new-moms-c-sections-without-consent.

Redhead, C. Stephen and Dabrowska, Agata. "Public health service agencies: Overview and funding (FY2010-FY2016)." U.S. Congressional Research Service. October 13, 2015. https://fas.org/sgp/crs/misc/R43304.pdf.

Reynolds, Mark. "Why Kate lied about Mia's birth." *Daily Mail* N.d. Accessed November 20, 2020. https://www.dailymail.co.uk/tvshowbiz/article-300032/Why -Kate-lied-Mias-birth.html.

Robertson, Patty. "Career information: Obstetrics and gynecology." *University of California – San Francisco School of Medicine.* April 2013. Accessed July 10, 2020. https://meded.ucsf.edu/md-program/current-students/resources-current -students/advising-and-career-development/career-advisors/career-information- obstetrics-gynecology.

Rogers, Ann E., Wei-Ting Hwang, Linda D. Scott, Linda H. Aiken, and David F. Dinges. "The working hours of hospital staff nurses and patient safety." *Health Affairs* 23, no. 4 (2004): 202–212.

Rooks, Judith Pence. *Midwifery and Childbirth in America.* Philadelphia, PA: Temple University Press, 1997.

Rosenthal, Elizabeth. *An American Sickness: How Healthcare Became Big Business and How You Can Take it Back.* New York: Penguin Press, 2017.

Roth, Louise Marie, and Megan M. Henley. "Unequal motherhood: Racial-ethnic and socioeconomic disparities in cesarean sections in the United States." *Social Problems* 59, no. 2 (2012): 207–227.

Roth, Louise Marie; Nicole Heidbreder, Megan M. Henley, Marla, Marek, Miriam Naiman-Sessions, Jennifer, Torres, and Christine H. Morton. "Maternity Support Survey: A Report on the Criss-National Surveys of Doulas, Childbirth Educators and Labor and Delivery Nurses in the United States and Canada." May 1, 2014. Accessed September 29, 2020. https://maternitysurvey.files.wordpress.com/2014/0 7/mss-report-5-1-14-final.pdf.

Rural Health Information Hub. "Critical Access Hospitals." Accessed November 17, 2020, https://www.ruralhealthinfo.org/topics/critical-access-hospitals.

Samuelson, Kristin W. "Post-traumatic stress disorder and declarative memory functioning: A review." *Dialogues in Clinical Neuroscience* 13, no. 3 (2011): 346–351.

Schiller, Rebecca. *Why Human Rights in Childbirth Matter.* London: Pinter and Martin, 2017.

Schniederjan, Stephanie, and G. Kevin Donovan. "Ethics versus education: Pelvic exams on anesthetized women." *The Journal of the Oklahoma State Medical Association* 98, no. 8 (2005): 386–388.

Scholten, Catherine M. "On the importance of the obstetrick art: Changing customs of childbirth in America, 1760–1825." In *Women and Health in America: Historical Readings*, edited by Judith Walzer Leavitt, 426–445 Madison, WI: University of Wisconsin Press, 1984.

Sears, Martha and William Sears. *The Attachment Parenting Book.* Boston: Little Brown and Company, 2001.

Sewell, Jane Eliot. *Cesarean Section – A Brief History.* Bethesda, MD: National Library of Medicine, 1993. https://www.nlm.nih.gov/exhibition/cesarean/index. html.

Shepherd-Banigan, Megan, and Janice F Bell. "Paid leave benefits among a national sample of working mothers with infants in the United States." *Maternal and Child Health Journal* 18, no. 1 (2014): 286–295, DOI:10.1007/s10995-013-1264-3.

Siegler, Kirk. "The struggle to hire and keep doctors in rural areas means patients go without care." *National Public Radio.* May 21, 2019. Accessed July 9, 2020. https://www.npr.org/sections/health-shots/2019/05/21/725118232/the-struggle-to -hire-and-keep-doctors-in-rural-areas-means-patients-go-without-c.

Silberner, Joanne. "Report: World support for mental health care is 'pitifully small'" *NPR.* October 15, 2018. Accessed November 8, 2020. https://www.npr.org/secti

ons/goatsandsoda/2018/10/15/656669752/report-world-support-for-mental-health-care-is-pitifully-small.

Simcox, Louise; Laura Ormesher, Clare Tower, and Ian Greer. "Pulmonary thrombo-embolism in pregnancy: diagnosis and management." *Breathe* 11, no. 4 (2015): 282–289.

Simpson, Kathleen Rice. "An overview of distribution of births in United States hospitals in 2008 with implications for small volume perinatal units in rural hospitals." *Journal of Obstetric, Gynecologic & Neonatal Nursing* 40, no. 4 (2011): 432–439.

Simpson, Madeleine, and Christine Catling. "Understanding psychological traumatic birth experiences: A literature review." *Women and Birth* 29, no. 3 (2016): 203–207.

Sinclair, Dana, and Lynne Murray. "Effects of postnatal depression on children's adjustment to school." *The British Journal of Psychiatry* 172, no. 1 (1998): 58–63.

Sit, Dorothy, Anthony J. Rothschild, and Katherine L. Wisner. "A review of postpartum psychosis." *Journal of Women's Health* 15, no. 4 (2006): 352–368.

Smith, Jeffrey Michael, Richard F. Lowe, Judith Fullerton, Sheena M. Currie, Laura Harris, and Erica Felker-Kantor. "An integrative review of the side effects related to the use of magnesium sulfate for pre-eclampsia and eclampsia management." *BMC Pregnancy and Childbirth* 13, no. 1 (2013): 34.

Sorenson, Dianna Spies, and Lois Tschetter. "Prevalence of negative birth perception, disaffirmation, perinatal trauma symptoms, and depression among postpartum women." *Perspectives in Psychiatric Care* 46, no. 1 (2010): 14–25.

Spear, Rachel N. "'Let Me Tell You a Story' on teaching trauma narratives, writing, and healing." *Pedagogy: Critical Approaches to Teaching Literature, Language, Composition, and Culture* 14, no. 1 (2014): 53–79.

Starkley, Adam. "Kate Hudson hit with backlash after saying having a c-section was 'lazy.'" Metro. September 14, 2017. https://metro.co.uk/2017/09/14/kate-hudson-hit-with-backlash-after-saying-having-a-c-section-was-lazy-6928815/.

Starr, Paul. "The social transformation of American medicine." PhD diss., Harvard University, 1978.

Stephenson, Joan. "Mental disorders undertreated." *Jama* 283, no. 3 (2000): 325–325.

Stone, Rebecca. "Pregnant women and substance use: Fear, stigma, and barriers to care." *Health Justice* 3, no. 2 (2015).

Substance Abuse and Mental Health Services Administration. "Key substance use and mental health indicators in the United States: Results from the 2017 National Survey on Drug Use and Health" (HHS Publication No. SMA 18-5068, NSUDH Series H-53). Rockville, MD: Center for Behavioral Health Statistics and Quality, Substance Abuse and Mental Health Services Administration. Retrieved from https://www.samhsa.gov/data/sites/default/files/cbhsq-reports/NSDUHFFR 2017/NSDUHFFR2017.pdf.

Sukel, Kayt. "Dealing with the shortage of rural physicians." *Medical Economics, August* 29 (2019).

Tajima-Peña, Renee. *No Más Bebés*, 2015.

Tamkin, Emily. "Finland's health-care system is ranked among the best in the world. Someone Tell Nikki Haley." *The Washington Post*. March 21, 2019. Accessed June 6, 2020. https://www.washingtonpost.com/world/2019/03/21/finlands-health-care-system-is-ranked-among-best-world-someone-tell-nikki-haley/.

Tarkka, Marja-Terttu, Marita Paunonen, and Pekka Laippala. "Social support provided by public health nurses and the coping of first-time mothers with child care." *Public Health Nursing* 16, no. 2 (1999): 114–119.

Texas Children's Hospital. "Recognizing signs of postpartum anxiety." Accessed November 20, 2020. https://women.texaschildrens.org/blog/recognizing-signs-postpartum-anxiety.

Thangamuthu, A., I. F. Russell, and M. Purva. "Epidural failure rate using a standardized definition." *International Journal of Obstetric Anesthesia* 22, no. 4 (2013): 310–315.

The American College of Obstetricians and Gynecologists. "Magnesium Sulfate Use in Obstetrics." Committee Opinion Number 652. 2016. https://www.acog.org/Clinical-Guidance-and-Publications/Committee-Opinions/Committee-on-Obstetric-Practice/Magnesium-Sulfate-Use-in-Obstetrics.

The Mayo Clinic. "C-section." Accessed November 21, 2020. https://www.mayoclinic.org/tests-procedures/c-section/about/pac-20393655.

The Mayo Clinic. 2020. "Mastitis." Accessed November 5, 2020. https://www.mayoclinic.org/diseases-conditions/mastitis/symptoms-causes/syc-20374829.

The Mayo Clinic. 2020. "Mental health: Overcoming the stigma of mental illness." Accessed November 8, 2020. https://www.mayoclinic.org/diseases-conditions/mental-illness/in-depth/mental-health/art-20046477.

The Mayo Clinic. 2020. "Nonstress test." Accessed October 26, 2020. https://www.mayoclinic.org/tests-procedures/nonstress-test/about/pac-20384577.

The Mayo Clinic. 2020. "Postpartum depression." Accessed September 29, 2020. https://www.mayoclinic.org/diseases-conditions/postpartum-depression/symptoms-causes/syc-20376617.

The Mayo Clinic. "Pregnancy week by week." Accessed July 7, 2020. https://www.mayoclinic.org/healthy-lifestyle/pregnancy-week-by-week/in-depth/pregnancy/art-20046098.

The Physicians Foundation. "2018 Survey of America's Physicians." The Physicians Foundation. Accessed August 20, 2020. https://physiciansfoundation.org/wp-content/uploads/2018/09/physicians-survey-results-final-2018.pdf.

Townsend, Susan F. "Obstetric conflict: When fetal and maternal interests are at odds." *Pediatrics in Review* 32, no. 1 (2012): 33–36.

Treisman, Rachel. "Whistleblower Alleges 'Medical Neglect,' Questionable Hysterectomies of ICE Detainees." September 16, 2020. Accessed October 5, 2020. https://www.wbez.org/stories/whistleblower-alleges-medical-neglect-questionable-hysterectomies-of-ice-detainees/e5b12292-62d4-4df7-b12e-cc650e3f07d7.

U.S. Census Bureau, Urban and Rural Population: 1900-1990; Census 2000 Summary File 1 Table P002; 2010 Census Summary File 1 Table P2, A Century of Delineating a Changing Landscape: The Census Bureau's Urban and Rural Classification, 1910 to 2010.

U.S. Census Bureau. "Fast Facts – Idaho." 2019. Accessed October 26, 2020. https://www.census.gov/quickfacts/ID.

U.S. Census Bureau. "Quickfacts: Idaho." Accessed June 20, 2020. https://www.census.gov/quickfacts/fact/table/ID/PST045219.

U.S. Census Bureau. "Quickfacts: Washington." Accessed June 20, 2020. https://www.census.gov/quickfacts/WA.

United States Department of Labor. "Family and Medical Leave (FMLA)." Accessed November 5, 2020. https://www.dol.gov/general/topic/benefits-leave/fmla.

Unützer, Jürgen; Harbin, Henry; Schoenbaum, Michael; and Druss, Benjamin. "The collaborative care model: An approach for integrating physical and mental health care in Medicaid health homes." Advancing Integrated Mental Health Solutions, University of Washington. Accessed November 8, 2020. https://aims.uw.edu/sites/default/files/CMSBrief_2013.pdf.

Vesga-Lopez, Oriana, Carlos Blanco, Katherine Keyes, Mark Olfson, Bridget F. Grant, and Deborah S. Hasin. "Psychiatric disorders in pregnant and postpartum women in the United States." *Archives of General Psychiatry* 65, no. 7 (2008): 805–815.

Virtanen, Marianna, Tiina Kurvinen, Kirsi Terho, Tuula Oksanen, Reijo Peltonen, Jussi Vahtera, Marianne Routamaa, Marko Elovainio, and Mika Kivimäki. "Work hours, work stress, and collaboration among ward staff in relation to risk of hospital-associated infection among patients." *Medical Care* (2009): 310–318.

Wagenfeld-Heintz Ellen, Victoria C. Ross and Keon-Hyung Lee. "Physicians' perceptions of patients in a county sponsored health plan." *Social Work in Public Health* 23, no. 1 (2007): 45–59, DOI: 10.1300/J523v23n01_03.

Waitzkin, Howard, and Holly Magana. "The black box in somatization: unexplained physical symptoms, culture, and narratives of trauma." *Social Science & Medicine* 45, no. 6 (1997): 811–825.

Wamsley, Laurel. "Finland's women-led government had equalized family leave." February 5, 2020. Accessed February 13, 2021. https://www.npr.org/2020/02/05/803051237/finlands-women-led-government-has-equalized-family-leave-7-months-for-each-parent.

Warland, Jane, Alexander EP Heazell, Tomasina Stacey, Christin Coomarasamy, Jayne Budd, Edwin A. Mitchell, and Louise M. O'Brien. "'They told me all mothers have worries,' stillborn mother's experiences of having a 'gut instinct' that something is wrong in pregnancy: Findings from an international case–control study." *Midwifery* 62 (2018): 171–176.

Waterbury, Jude T. "Refuting patients' obligations to clinical training: A critical analysis of the arguments for an obligation of patients to participate in the clinical education of medical students." *Medical Education* 35, no. 3 (2001): 286–294.

Weiss, Shimon, Eric Goldlust, and Yvonne Vaucher. "Improving parent satisfaction: An intervention to increase neonatal parent–provider communication." *Journal of Perinatology* 30, no. 6 (2010): 425–430.

Wen, Leana. "I'm Pregnant. What would happen if I couldn't afford health care?" NPR. March 11, 2017. Accessed May 24, 2020. https://www.npr.org/sections/health-shots/2017/03/11/519416036/im-pregnant-what-would-happen-if-i-couldnt-afford-health-care.

White, Robert D. "Individual rooms in the NICU—an evolving concept." *Journal of Perinatology* 23, no. 1 (2003): S22–S24.

White, Robert D., Judith A. Smith, and Mardelle M. Shepley. "Recommended standards for newborn ICU design." *Journal of Perinatology* 33, no. 1 (2013): S2–S16.

Williams, Caitlin R., Celeste Jerez, Karen Klein, Malena Correa, Jose Belizan, and Gabriela Cormick. "Obstetric violence: A Latin American legal response to mistreatment during childbirth." *An International Journal of Obstetrics and Gynaecology* 125, no. 10 (2018): 1208–1211.

Williams, Serena. "Serena Williams: What my life-threatening experience taught me about giving birth." *Cable News Network*. February 20, 2018. https://www.cnn.com/2018/02/20/opinions/protect-mother-pregnancy-williams-opinion/index.html.

Wilson, Reid. 2017. "Rural poverty skyrockets as jobs move away." *The Hill*. December 5, 2017. Accessed June 18, 2020. https://thehill.com/homenews/state-watch/363415-rural-poverty-skyrockets-as-jobs-move-away;

Wilson, Robin Fretwell. "Autonomy suspended: Using female patients to teach intimate exams without their knowledge or consent." *Journal of Health Care Law & Policy* 8, no. 2 (2005): 240–263.

Wolf, Jacqueline. *Cesarian Section*. Baltimore, MD: Johns Hopkins University Press, 2018.

World Health Organization. "Care in normal birth: A practical guide." *Birth* 24, no. 2 (1997).

World Health Organization. "Density of physicians." Accessed July 6, 2020. https://www.who.int/gho/health_workforce/physicians_density/en/.

World Health Organization. "Monitoring Emergency Obstetric Care." Accessed February 5, 2021. https://apps.who.int/iris/bitstream/handle/10665/44121/9789241547734_eng.pdf;jsessionid=19D4C0CF81B953E872746DF9A32FD7E4?sequence=1.

Wrate, R. M., A. C. Rooney, P. F. Thomas, and J. L. Cox. "Postnatal depression and child development: A three-year follow-up study." *The British Journal of Psychiatry* 146, no. 6 (1985): 622–627.

Yildiz, Pelin Dikmen, Susan Ayers, and Louise Phillips. "The prevalence of post-traumatic stress disorder in pregnancy and after birth: A systematic review and meta-analysis." *Journal of Affective Disorders* 208 (2017): 634–645.

Zhao, Lan. *Why Are Fewer Hospitals in the Delivery Business?* Bethesda, MD: NORC at the University of Chicago, 2007.

Index

About the Author

Kristin Haltinner is an associate professor of sociology at the University of Idaho.

www.ingramcontent.com/pod-product-compliance
Lightning Source LLC
Chambersburg PA
CBHW022317280326
41932CB00010B/1131